MAKEUP
THE ULTIMATE GUIDE

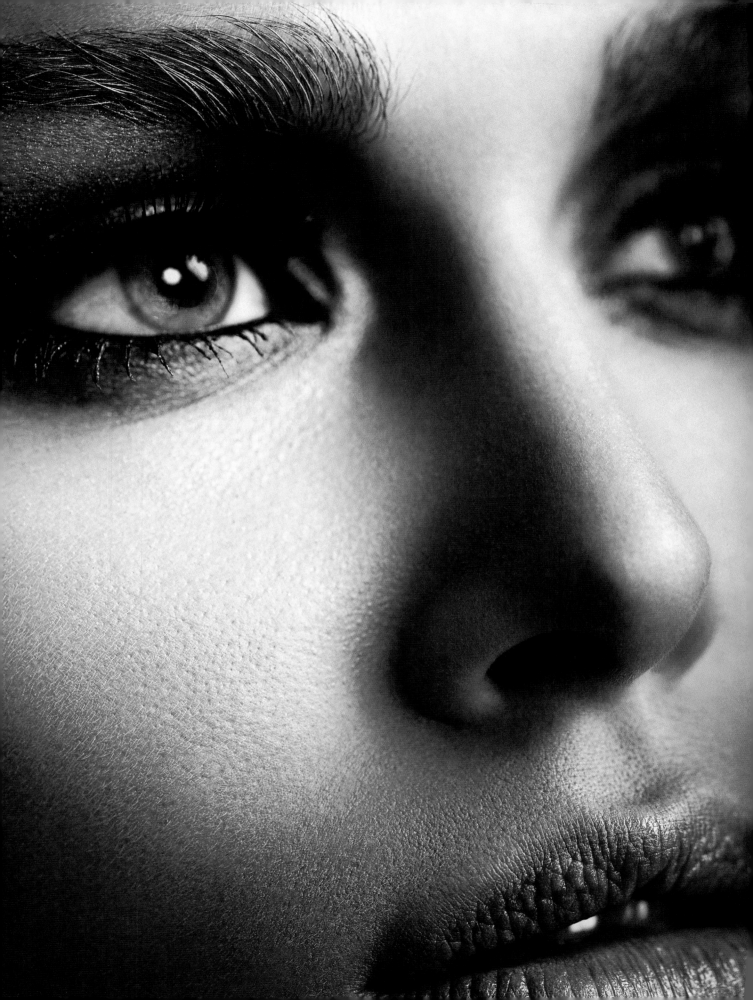

RAE MORRIS

MAKEUP
THE ULTIMATE GUIDE

Photography by Steven Chee

APPLE

First published in the UK in 2008 by Apple Press
Reprinted in 2008, 2009 (twice), 2010 (twice), 2011

Apple Press
7 Greenland Street
London NW1 0ND
United Kingdom
www.apple-press.com

Created and produced by Arena Books, an imprint of
Allen & Unwin Pty Ltd
83 Alexander Street
Crows Nest NSW 2065
Australia
Phone: (61 2) 8425 0100
Fax: (61 2) 9906 2218
Email: info@allenandunwin.com
Web: www.allenandunwin.com

All notations of errors or omissions should be addressed to Whitecap Books Ltd., Editorial
Department, at the above address. All other correspondence (author inquiries, permissions,
and rights) concerning the content of this book should be addressed to Allen & Unwin, 83
Alexander St. Crows Nest NSW 2065, Australia.

ISBN 978-1-84543-266-9

Cataloguing-in-Publication data available upon request

Design by Seymour Designs

Printed in China through Colorcraft Ltd, Hong Kong

dedication

This book would not be possible if Richard Sharah hadn't taught
me what I know today.

Richard, you are still my mentor and the best makeup artist that ever lived!
I feel so blessed, enriched and honoured to have been trained by you.

Thank you for teaching me everything you knew, and for passing on your knowledge
and talent, and making sure I learnt it all. Thank you for your guidance, inspiration
and your incredible discipline.

I will never forget what a great talent you were, and will listen
to your voice in my head forever.

I miss you and will always love you.

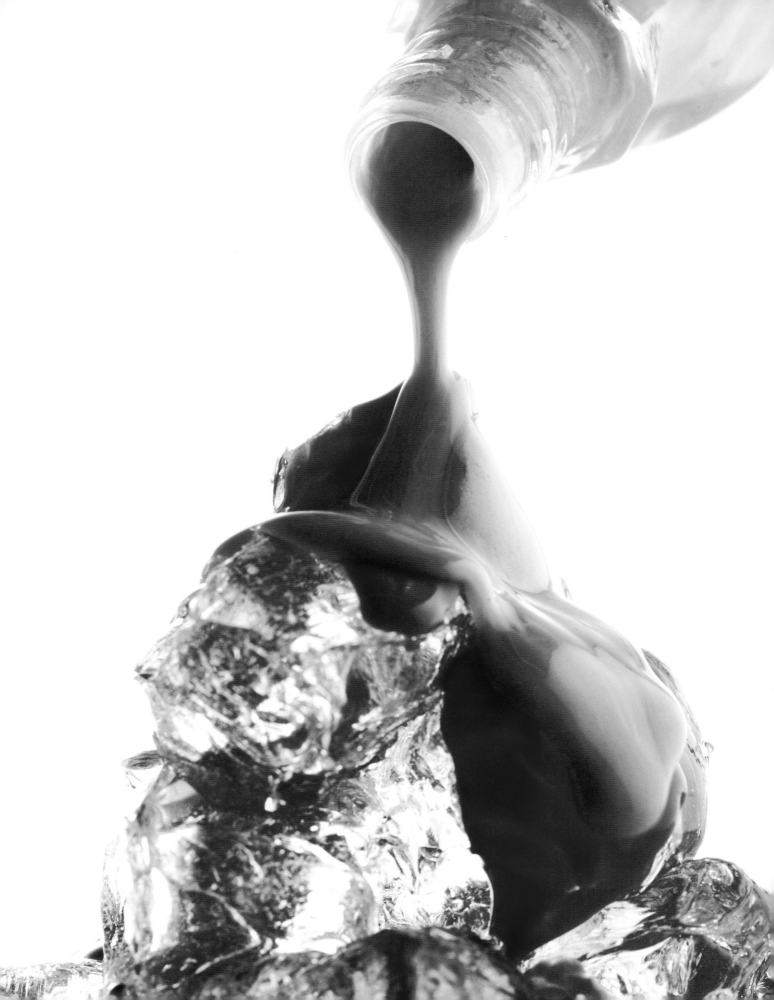

acknowledgements

I would like to say a huge thankyou to all those who helped make this book possible:

Alethea Gold, without whom none of this would be possible; Richard Sharah, my mentor; and Dotti.

Dolores Lavin - DLM, Ben Croft, Grace Testa - Studio Twenty4, Bronwyn Fraser (www.styleestablishment.com.au), Scott - ACMUSE, Maria - Makeup Store, Jo - MAC and Jodi Gardner.

Steven Chee, Katie Nolan, Dan Nadel, Kate Ursi and Matt.

My literary agents Mark Byrne and Lisa Hanrahan, and my publisher Jude McGee and editor Alexandra Nahlous.

My assistants Victoria Baron, Rachel Brook, Nicole Rossetto, Jane Drew, Ana Slavka, Sandra Cook, Nikki Halsted, Giorgi Ciot, Mandi Levanah - DLM, Martin Bray - The Artist Group, Cassie Sobel, and the students of Cameron Jane Makeup School.

Special thanks for the expert advice of Dr Van Park B.Sc. (Med). M.B.B.S., F.R.A.C.G.P. and Dr Peter L. Dixon M.B.B.S. F.R.A.C.S.

Stylists: Jennifer Smit - DLM, Michael Azzollini, Richard Milvain and Wil Ariyamethe - DLM.

Hair: Brad Ballard, Dario Cotroneo using GHD, Julianne McGuigan - DLM, Karen Hopwood - DLM, Lores Giglio - DLM, Michael Brennan - The Artist Group, Muriel Vancauwen - RP Represents www.rprepresents.com and Raymond Robinson - DLM.

Illustrators: Nigel Stanislaus and Dennis White.

Models: Abbey - Bella Model Management & Ford Models, New York, Ada - Chic Models, Alice - Chic Models, Annika - Chic Models, Bianca - Chic Models, Camille Piazza - Chic Models, Cassie - Chic Models, Catherine McNeil - Chic Models, Cheyenne Tozzi - Priscillas Model Management, Emma Booth - William Morris, Eunice Ward - Chadwick, Felicity King - Vivien's, Florence - Chic Models, Gemma Poole - Vivien's, Gemma Stooke - Priscillas Model Management, Jamie Moore - Scoop Management, Jodi Gardner - Chic Models, Kate Alstergren - Mark Byrne Management, Katie Lange - Chadwick, Kieta - Chic Models, Kirstie Penn - Chic Models, Kristine Duran - Chic Models, Lara Bingle, Lizzy B - Chic Models, Lucy Bayet - Chadwick, Michelle Leslie, Miranda Kerr - Chic Models, Olivia Dunnfrost - Chadwick, Renee Mansbridge - Chic Models, Sam Blades - Chic Models, Sarah Grant - Mark Byrne Management, Sonya Kukainis - Vivien's, Stephanie Carta - Chic Models, Tottie Goldsmith, Valerija - Chic Models, Ursula Hufnagl, Dr Van Park and Xiya Xu - Vivien's.

And finally, thank you to Dov for all the terrific catering, Echelon Studios, Justin Braitling - Location House, David and Melinda Itzkowic - Location House, Kellie Tissear, Francis Callanan, Jeremy Southern and John Williams.

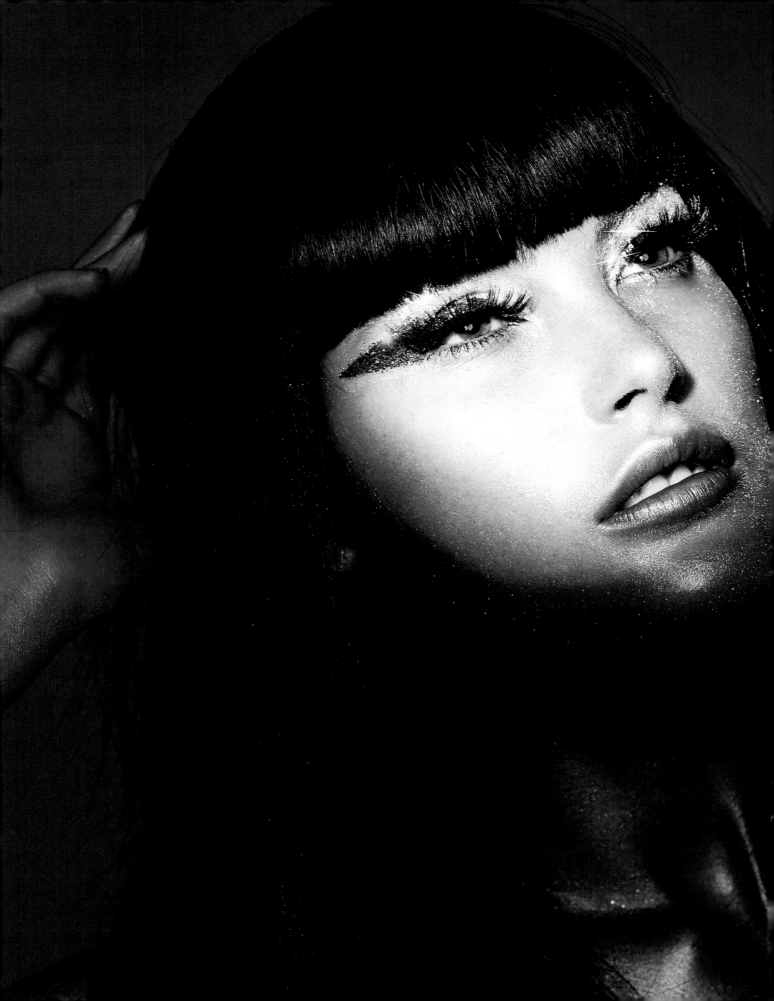

contents

I fell into makeup. Well, not literally, although I have done that too. What I mean is makeup crept up on me and took me by surprise. I started my working life as a hairdresser, and it was in this guise that I found myself at the Miss Model of the World pageant in Istanbul in 1993. There I was, quietly at work on a model's hair, little knowing that destiny, in the shapely form of Naomi Campbell, was about to rear its extremely beautiful head.

Naomi was on the other side of the room with a male makeup artist when, suddenly, there was a flurry of angry voices then he was heading for the door in a flood of tears. In the stunned silence that followed, Naomi glared around the room and fortunately (although it didn't feel that way at the time) her gaze fell on me. 'Fix my lips,' she said. I looked at her mouth, then at the lip gloss on the bench, then back to her mouth. A wave of completely unwarranted confidence swept over me and I thought, 'How hard can it be?'

Before I had the chance to talk myself out of it, I picked up the lip gloss and got to work with only moderately shaky hands. As I did, the door burst open and the whole room erupted in a blaze of flashlights. The paparazzi had arrived … Next thing I knew, my picture was plastered all over the tabloids and my makeup career had officially begun. So before I go on, I'd like to say a belated thanks to Naomi for the dummy spit that made all this possible.

Fast-forward fifteen years and I now find myself writing a book. And I suppose the important question is, 'What makes this book any different from all the others that are out there?' Well, first of all, this book is designed to bring high-end fashion makeup into the realm of everyday life and into the hands of the everyday consumer. Every single look (even the most glamorous one) has a simple step-by-step photo guide and clear, concise instructions to help even the most inexperienced beginner apply the makeup.

The looks I have chosen are not crazy fashion fads that are going to be out of style this time next year, nor are they boring brown and beige tones. All the looks in this book have been chosen because they are glamorous, sexy and, above all, *timeless*. And, for the first time, you will find out all the sneaky tricks that we makeup artists use when buying makeup. I've held nothing back! And over the coming pages you will learn how to tell the difference between a good product and a crap one.

Another thing I've aimed to do is to teach you makeup in exactly the same way that I do it and teach my assistants and students. I've included all the simple, practical tips, time-saving measures and shortcuts (or cheats, if you like) that I employ on a daily basis, to achieve those amazing results you see in magazines. So not only have I tried and tested them all, I've made them super-easy to follow.

Remember, just like any technique, makeup requires practice. If you don't get it right the first time round, don't stress. I have been doing it for years and I still have to wipe it all off and start again from time to time. So pick up your brushes, your lipsticks and your blushes and practise, practise, practise. And don't forget to have fun with it!

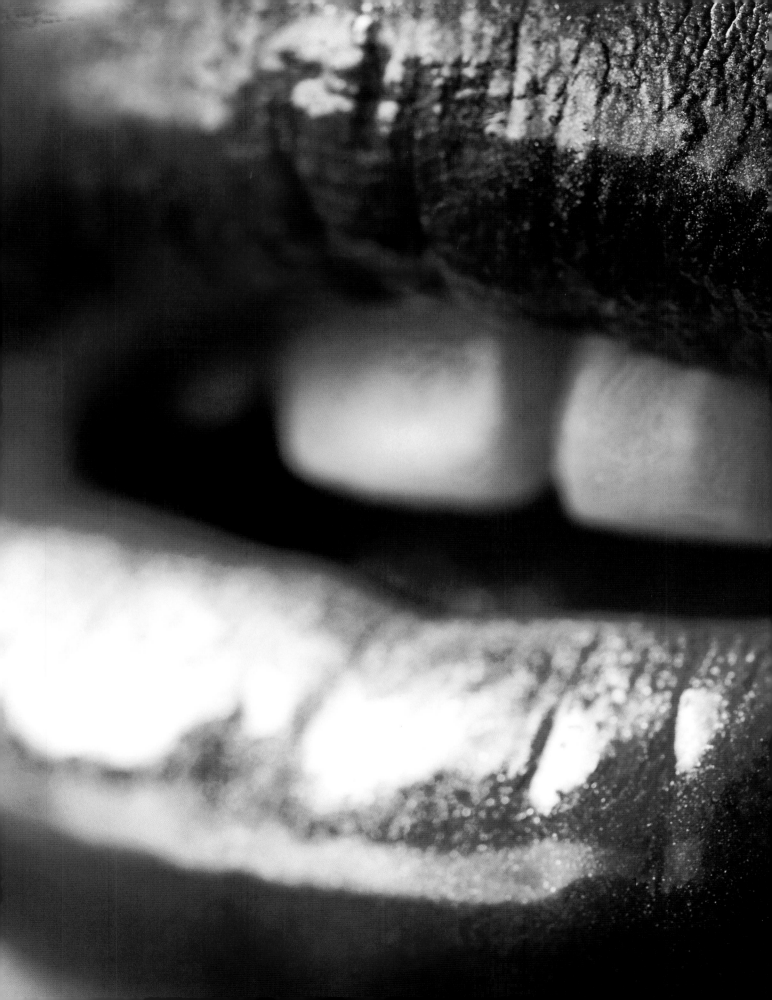

¹essentials

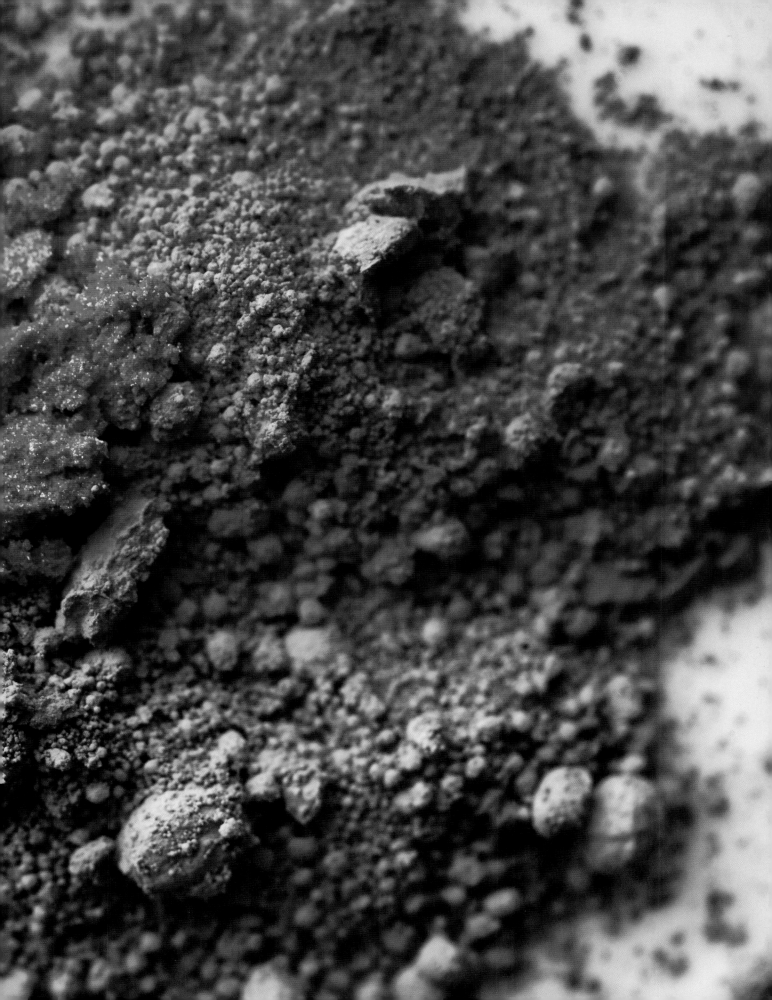

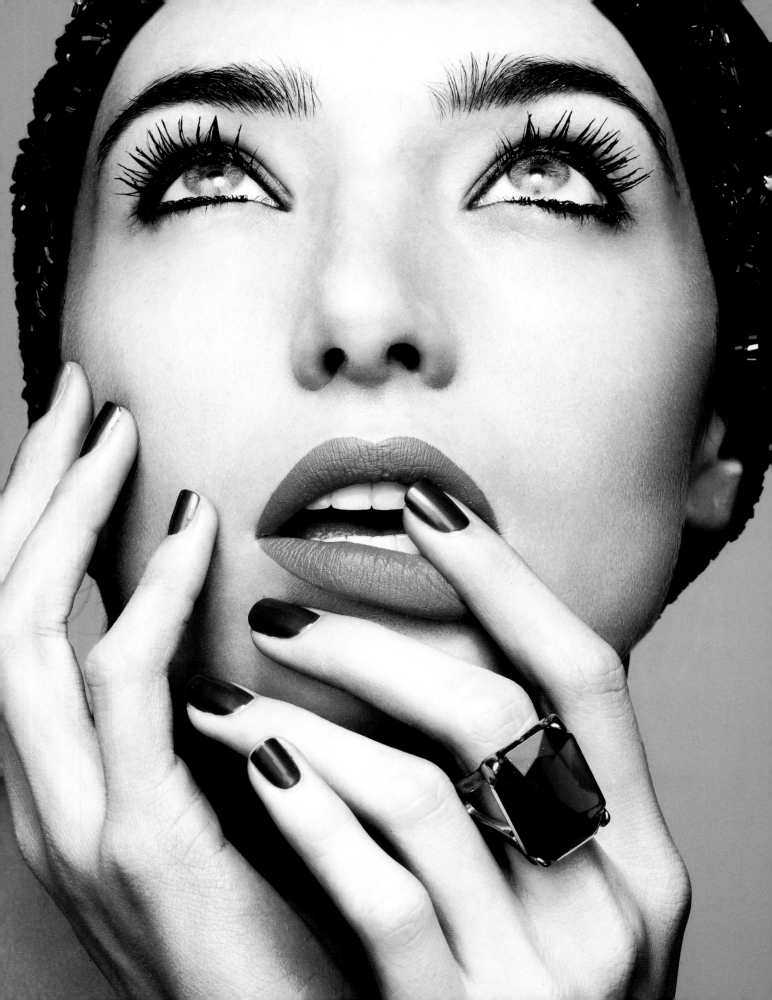

makeup kit

You would never see a makeup artist backstage at Paris Fashion Week with a few cotton buds and a couple of sponge-tip applicators. That's because to do the right makeup, you need the right makeup tools.

The correct tools make the job easier, and they give you the control for doing your makeup properly. That's why, when it comes to makeup, you really are only as good as the tools you use!

Because I travel a lot, my makeup is constantly damaged, but knowing I have my brushes, for example, makes it okay because I can always run to buy new makeup—I can even use what's in a model's bag—but I can't round up brushes in an emergency.

I know that I couldn't do my job without my tools, so I have compiled a list of what I believe are ESSENTIALS for you to own in your very own makeup kit. Yes, it is a bit longer than you might like it to be, but too bad! Believe me when I tell you, it's an investment and worth every cent. Most of the items listed will last you for years, some even a lifetime. One way to keep costs down is to spend less on disposable items such as lipstick and eye shadow, to make way for the more necessary things like brushes.

Because brushes are incredibly important, I've added a whole section on them, explaining the different types available and how to use them (see pages 10–15).

But first, let's begin with what you need for your makeup kit.

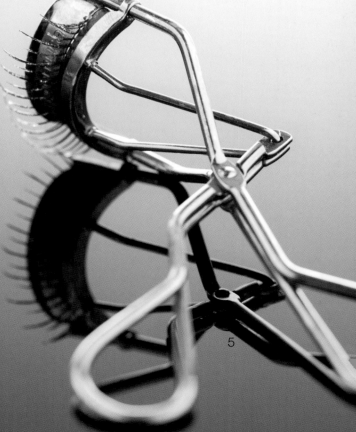

Two to three eye shadows

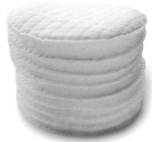

I know women with hundreds, but you can achieve a lot with just two. To know which colours you should choose, see the Eye Colour Charts chapter (page 42). When you're at the makeup counter and you spot a colour you love, you can do the 'one wipe trick' to test the product. Take a clean fingertip, wipe over the product once, and look at the intensity. If the colour isn't as intense on your finger as it looks like in the package, then don't buy it—you'll be forever trying to build up that colour on your eye. It's better to have a colour that's strong and you can soften with loose translucent powder. Also, watch out for dodgy multicoloured pigments. After the 'one wipe trick', grab a cotton bud and lightly dust your finger to see what colour you're left with. This is great for testing deep metallic eye shadows such as ruby-reds and dark blues. If the product is bad, then rubbing with the bud will wipe away all the rich colour and leave you only with the black.

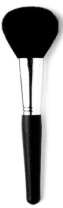

Brushes

Absolutely essential! You are going to need several of these, so I've included a thorough list on pages 10–15.

Black mascara

To be used with a clean wand or comb on standby.

Cotton pads

Use for applying powder. I prefer these because most powder brushes leave brush marks. Powder brushes and buffs need to be cleaned so often that maintenance becomes a hassle—cotton pads are a great replacement and the most hygienic option.

Bicarb of soda

For prepping the skin. You can use this once a week as an exfoliant—bicarb is the best exfoliant you can ever use. Pour a tablespoon into your hands, and mix with a water-based cleanser (Cetaphil is my favourite) until you get a gritty texture (like a scrub). Apply as you would normally use an exfoliant, then wash your face. Don't use if you have chemical peels of any kind, if you are sunburnt or are using AHA, BHA, retinols or any acne-related medications—these products make your skin peel chemically, so there's no need to re-scrub with an exfoliant.

Makeup primer

Makeup primers are basically a moisturiser that contains extra silicone and glycerin, allowing foundation to be applied a lot more evenly. If you use a makeup primer don't use a moisturiser as you would be doubling up—let your makeup primer act as your moisturiser as well.

Black pencil

This should not be waterproof so that it can be applied inside the eye for those glamorous occasions. This works well as smudged eyeliner on the top lash line. If the weather is cold, you should heat up your pencil before using it, by rubbing it on the back of your hand, to release the pigment and soften the pencil; this should give it a crayon-like feel and improve the intensity of the colour.

Tweezers

Pointed tweezers are my favourite because they remove every hair in sight, and they outline the brow beautifully. However, because they are like needles, you must turn the tweezers side on, rather than directly pointing them at the brow.

Inner eye white pencil

To clean up redness in the inner rim of the eye. This opens the eye and makes you look instantly younger and more awake. Make sure that it's not waterproof as the inner rim is wet!

Brow pencil

Use one that matches your brow hair colour, not what you wish it to be.

Highlighter

Use one that matches your skin tone. See the Highlighting chapter on page 194.

Cream blush

This is great if you don't like to use powder of any kind. It gives a more creamy, dewy finish to the cheeks, which provides a youthful look. Don't use cream blush if you have powdered your foundation.

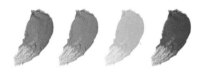

Cream, liquid or gel eyeliner in black

I love the creams; they give you time to blend and when they dry they don't move or smudge, plus most of them are waterproof. They come in awesome shades such as blue-black, bronze and turquoise.

Eyelash curlers

This is the one tool I believe every woman must own. Professionals use them *every single* time and so should you. There is a simple trick to them: place your lashes in the curlers, then slightly squeeze the curlers before you start, making sure there is no skin trapped, then squeeze as hard as you can for 5 to 10 seconds before releasing. You can also buy heated curlers, which are easier to use. These are battery operated, and you can also heat them up with a hairdryer if the battery goes flat. If you do heat up with a hairdryer, please check how hot they are on another part of your face, such as the chin, before going near the eye. Heated curlers are particularly good to use for upkeep, after applying mascara; curling lashes with standard curlers after mascara has been applied can result in clumps.

Translucent powder

Even if you hate powder, you'll need this for blending and prepping your eyes. Beware of any powder that has titanium dioxide (even though it's essential for sunscreen); it's completely safe for everyday use, however, it will play havoc if you're going to a special occasion where a camera flash may be involved. The reason for this is that titanium (in its pure form) will photograph pure white, so if it's in your powder it can whiten your foundation by up to five shades. On the other hand, titanium has great sunscreen benefits.

At least two foundations

These are a must, especially if you use a fake tan, and if your skin changes colour from summer to winter.

Concealer

Speaks for itself; necessary for anyone with discolouration, blemishes, bags, pigmentation, etc.

Contouring cream or shadow

For shading purposes (to build cheekbones etc). It's not for everyone, but it makes one hell of a difference. See the Contouring chapter on page 158 for more information.

Lip gloss and lipstick

Again, you don't need hundreds, and if you own hundreds, squash them into a palette (you can get them cheap from haberdashery shops—they're called 'bobbin cases'—or you can buy cheap empty palettes from makeup stores). However, I believe every woman should own a clear and a tinted lip gloss, a great nude shade (that makes your lips bigger), a gold or shimmery gloss highlighter (which you will see I use extensively throughout this book), and your signature colour. Remember, lipsticks go off; you can tell by the sudden smell or taste change. And, yes, every woman can wear red lipstick!

Gold or silver shimmer powder (pigments)

These are used to highlight the eyes, the cheeks and the lips. They give the skin a glow, and bring your makeup alive. Gold is for warm-toned skins and silver is for cool-toned skins. In this book I have used these pigments in almost every shot.

Powder blush

This is the blush to use if you have powdered your foundation—powder on powder blends. Only use powder blush if you have powdered your skin with translucent powder after applying your foundation otherwise it will have a blotchy and uneven effect. Not all powder blushes are matt. My favourite kind is that which has a gold shimmer to give an extra glow.

brushes

It constantly amazes me that week in week out, I see women attempting to do their face with just one brush. But even a top makeup artist can't do great makeup with only one brush, so how can you? The truth is that you are going to need many brushes, and yes, that is going to cost a bit. I spend a fortune on brushes every year and I've often wished I could just buy a cheap one and be done with it. But I simply can't. I have to have the right equipment, and so do you.

How to choose the good-quality—not necessarily expensive—brushes

I'm going to let you in on one of the best kept secrets in buying makeup brushes, and it's so simple. Whenever you want to buy a makeup brush, balance it on its very tip. Hold the brush vertically on the back of your hand, bristles down, and lightly bounce the brush to test the strength of the bristles. The bristles should only have a slight bend; if they splay, or flatten completely, then the brush will be too difficult to use, and the makeup will go everywhere except where you want to put it.

When you are doing detailed work such as applying eyeliner or defining a brow, you need to add a little pressure with your brush as you apply it. If you have a bad brush, the slightest pressure will move the bristles from 1 mm to (if it's really nasty) 5 mm. That is a huge distance when you are talking about an eyeliner.

And from spending years looking at brushes from all around the world across all different price ranges, I still find my kit consists of the cheapest to the most expensive—it's about a 50/50 ratio. So you can and will find brushes that are in your price range; check out discount makeup stores, art and craft shops and manchester stores.

How to clean your brushes

The best way to clean your brushes is with brush cleaner once a week. However, if you don't have brush cleaner, try hot, soapy water—I actually use washing detergent; shampoo probably isn't strong enough. Under hot, soapy water, rub your brush on a white plate. This way, when you clean your brush, you can see the colour on the plate. When the plate is clean and the water runs clear, you know the brush is washed. Then just let it dry overnight.

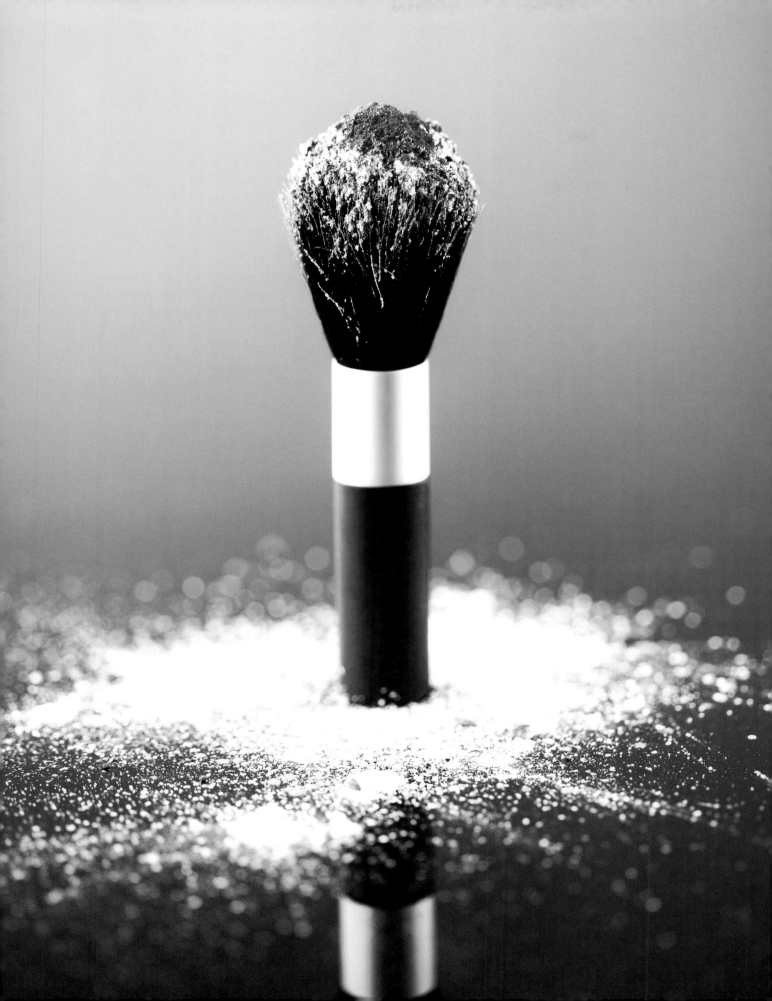

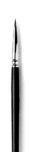

Fine-tip eyeliner brush

This is terrific for fine eyeliner. As it is delicate in nature, it has a limited life. I typically buy one every eight to twelve weeks, so you will have to replace it regularly. To get the most value out of this brush, look for a quality inexpensive one. You'd be surprised what you can find in an art supplies store. Sometimes I buy liquid eyeliner just for the brush as they are so firm. (I am also finding the new fine felt-tip eyeliner pens fantastic.) Remember, you don't have to use the product the brush comes with; I use them with a variety of other products as they give such a precise line and they last for ages. Besides using this brush for fine eyeliner, it's very useful for micro-concealing, adding highlights or diamond dust to the inner corners of the eyes, and embedding eye shadow right into the eyelash line to ensure there are no gaps.

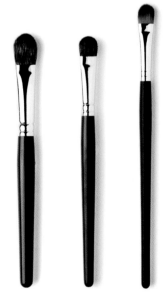

Large- and medium-sized rounded eye-shadow brushes

Notice I said rounded? That's because these brushes have to blend and move with your natural eye contours. Square brushes speak for themselves: they are 'square' so they give hard, unblended edges.

Small-sized rounded eye-shadow brush/concealer brush

This is exactly the same shape as your large- and medium-sized brushes, only it's downsized. As a makeup artist, I cannot work without one. I use it when working with intense pigments, for adding socket lines, or when working close to the eyelash line. It also doubles as a great concealer brush; just make sure you clean it in between uses.

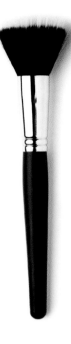

Fibre-optic foundation brush

Thank goodness for technology! I have yet to come across a more fantastic brush than the fibre-optic foundation brush. It makes any foundation application look flawless, even airbrushed at times. You can use this brush with all types of foundation. A word of warning, though: the white-tip bristles are extremely porous and will hold a lot of foundation, so the best way to use the brush is to apply the foundation to your face directly then use the brush to blend. If you are using the brush to absorb liquid foundation straight from the bottle, be mindful of how much foundation the brush will carry because you might end up with too much foundation on your face. Does wall paint ring a bell? Here's a great tip to avoid this: only allow about a quarter of the brush to be immersed in your foundation. You can always apply more if this isn't quite enough. You can also apply the foundation to the back of your hand and pick it up from there.

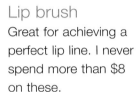

Lip brush

Great for achieving a perfect lip line. I never spend more than $8 on these.

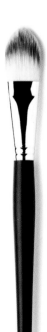

Flat foundation brush

This was the predecessor to the fibre-optic brush, and it is still a fantastic tool that will never date. This brush has many uses, namely for contouring, shading or highlighting using cream-based products, and is particularly great for cleaning up eye-shadow fallout from underneath the eye. Use this brush to apply foundation beneath the eye after completing a strong smoky eyes look, for example, as sometimes the bristles of the fibre-optic brush can run over the eye area and make a mess of the eye shadow.

Fine-tip brush

This is great for concealing and for using under the eyes, and for liquid eyeliner.

13

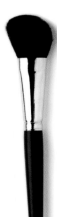

Contouring brush

This is very useful for contouring, which can make you look ten years younger.

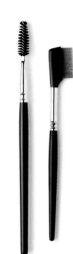

Mascara wand and metal comb

Mascara wands are available from all good makeup outlets, but you can also use your old mascara wand (please wash it first). I use this every single time after I apply mascara to comb out clumps and evenly spread out lashes. It's also great for eyebrows. Here's a little trick: spray the wand with hairspray before using on your brows and it will keep them in place. **Second choice:** Metal comb. I love these but I have seen a few accidents where women have stabbed themselves in the eye, so please use carefully. This is the best tool for combing up eyebrows.

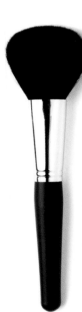

Blush brush

Most times you can use your contouring brush (I buy these from pharmacies— no need for an expensive one).

Fine angled brush

This is an essential brush. There isn't a woman on the planet who doesn't need this one! It's a must for eyebrows as it fills them in perfectly and allows you to extend your brows successfully. It's also one of the best brushes to do every kind of eyeliner imaginable. **Second choice:** There isn't one!

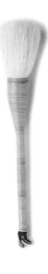

Kabuki

My favourite! This brush is a must-have. It's cheap and a little hard to find because it comes directly from Japan. However, some makeup wholesalers or distributors will get it for you. This brush is like a ball of cotton wool. It gives the smoothest finish and can be used for powder, all types of blush and bronzer, contouring and shading, and for blending eye shadow. **Second choice:** If you can't find a kabuki brush, you can use a rounded blush brush (i.e. not flat or cut straight).

Brush cleaner

Some of the products out there are laughable; I don't want my brushes to have deep-conditioning treatments, be oiled or smell like roses. I want to know that if I am working on a model with a cold sore or if I drop my brush on the floor, when I dip that brush into my cleaner it is going to kill all bacteria to a hospital grade, INSTANTLY. Sure, it smells like pure alcohol and the fumes can make your eyes water for a few seconds, but it's only momentary as an alcohol-based cleaner dries in seconds. Conversely, your conditioning cleaners will stay wet and the brushes will have a greasy film, which makes them a nightmare to work with. A good brush cleaner will clean a filthy brush instantly, with the brush drying in seconds, ready for its next use. You won't find a good makeup artist without a brush cleaner. Again, they are not the easiest to find, but you can ask your local makeup wholesaler to purchase it; the good news is that a litre of brush cleaner won't break the bank. Some cosmetic companies do sell their own brush cleaners; my advice is to test it first: it should dry within 10 seconds without leaving an oily film.

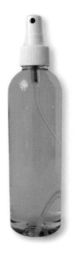

²skin prepping

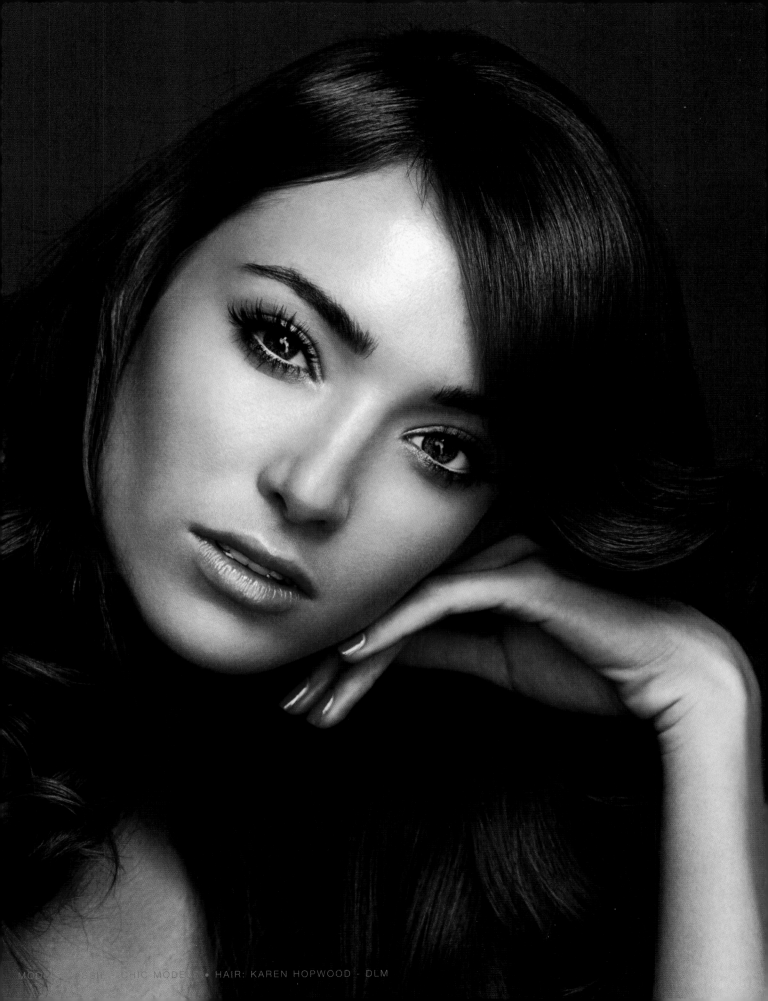

introduction to skin prepping

This book is not about skincare—that is a whole other complicated subject that we don't need to go into. So when it comes to prepping your skin, I'm going to cut to the chase.

I work with a different skin type every single day, but I don't have the time or kit size to carry every single cosmetic product available. I use the same products on everyone; the only things that change are whether or not I need sunscreen (we spend a lot of time inside a studio), choosing between an oil-based and water-based moisturiser (depending on the foundation I need to use, and if the skin is oily I don't use one at all—most of us forget how much moisturiser there is in foundation already!), and whether or not I need to use a toner (I do if the skin is extra oily or sometimes just in the eyelids as this area can get so greasy!).

Having said this, I ensure that all the products I use are perfume-free and can cause no reactions. I research every single product that goes into my kit and my philosophy is, if you can't use it on sunburnt or recently lasered skin, I won't use it at all.

But before you can even think about applying makeup, you need to prep your skin properly. If skin isn't prepped before I commence makeup, I actually can't apply it. And it's so easy to do. In emergencies it can be done in less than 20 seconds!

Remember, if you have an uneven skin texture to start with you'll have an uneven makeup to finish with, so take note of the step-by-step skin-prepping instructions on the following pages.

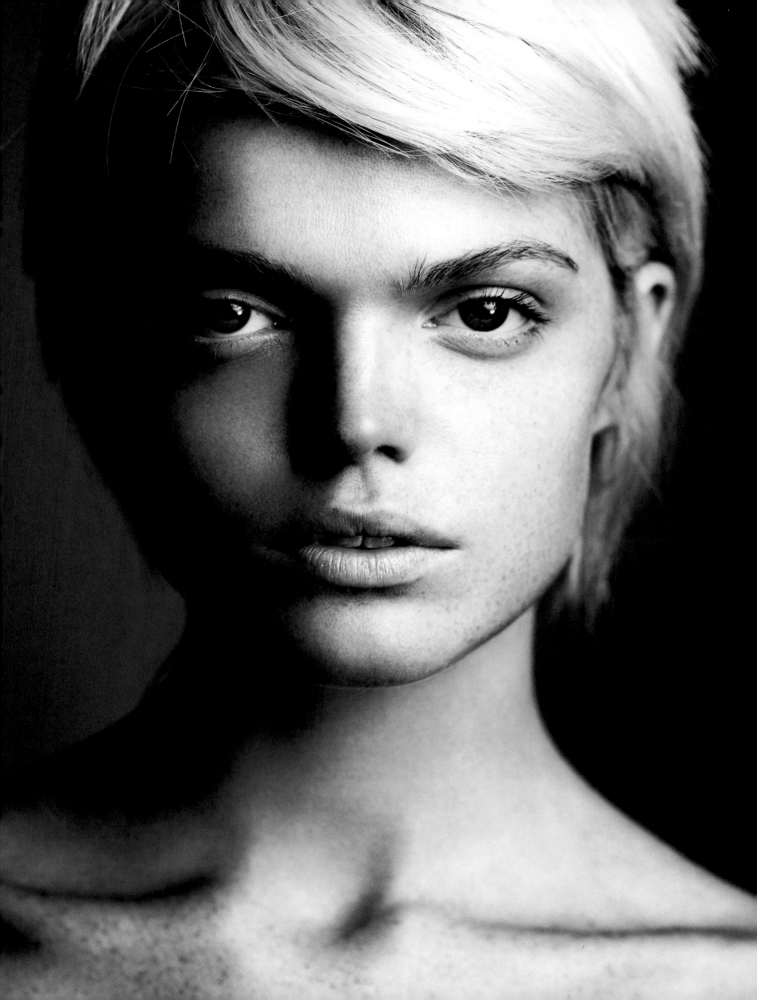

step-by-step skin prep

First thing's first: are you using water- or oil-based foundation and moisturiser? It's important to know this because you need an even canvas to begin with. The simple fact is that if you're using an oil-based moisturiser, it won't mix with a water-based foundation. Basic science, really. So check that all your products (concealer included) are either all water-based or all oil-based. This is the biggest reason why makeup won't last and yet it's the last thing most women would think about.

Step 1
Cleanse your skin with a pH-balanced product; it's important that you use nothing that leaves a film.

Step 2
Use a toner if you insist; I don't always use them, but they do come in handy when you just need to remove excess oil, or if you're going out and there is no time to wash your face. Just load up cotton pads and go for it; they will cleanse the skin surprisingly well. You need to check that your toner doesn't leave a residue as it will affect your makeup.

Step 3
Moisturise or use a primer, but remember, you don't need both. If you pile on two or three layers of cream, your makeup will slide—another basic fact. Don't moisturise your eyelids—I explain this in the eye-prepping step-by-steps opposite. And make sure at least one of your products contains sunscreen.

Two-minute emergency skin prep
This is for those quick-fix situations where you can't rinse your skin or there's no toner in sight. Wipe your face with alcohol-free and perfume-free baby wipes. Don't use glamorous cosmetic makeup wipes as they are designed to remove your makeup and they leave a creamy removal residue. This would be the equivalent of putting nail polish over nail polish remover—it won't allow your makeup to blend over your skin.

step-by-step eye prep

Most women don't realise that the eyelids are one of the oiliest parts of the face. If you don't believe me, go ahead and wipe your eyelids. You will find the same kind of oil you would find in your T-zone.

Oil is the number one killer of eye shadow. So all oil must be removed from your eyelids before applying eye shadow. The only time I don't remove oil is when I want greasy eyes for a photo shoot.

If you have some doubts about this, try this little experiment. Prep one eye according to the steps below, and then apply eye shadow. Then apply eye shadow to your other eye as you would normally do, without prepping, and watch the difference in the way your eye makeup lasts on your prepped eye. I never retouch eye makeup, even on a twelve-hour shoot, because I always prep the eyes properly.

Step 1

Cleanse your lids with a water-based cleanser. You can also use alcohol- and perfume-free baby wipes—that's what I use on every shoot. Do not moisturise your eyelids afterwards.

Step 2

The biggest question: do I apply foundation to the eyelids or don't I? My answer is yes, absolutely, every single time. Why? Because your eyelids, if you look closely at them, have blue and red tones or tinges. When you apply foundation, you knock out all the blue–red tones, giving you a great neutral canvas to allow your eye shadows to be true to their colour. (To test the true colour of your eye shadow, particularly if it's your favourite, apply a swatch of it to the back of your hand, and another swatch to your fingertip. And look at the difference in colour.) And remember, all foundations contain a moisturiser of some kind. This is all the moisture you will need on your eyelids.

Step 3

Lightly powder the eyelids with translucent powder. You can do this with a cotton pad. Powder will go cakey (not what you want) if you have too much oil or moisturiser on your lids.

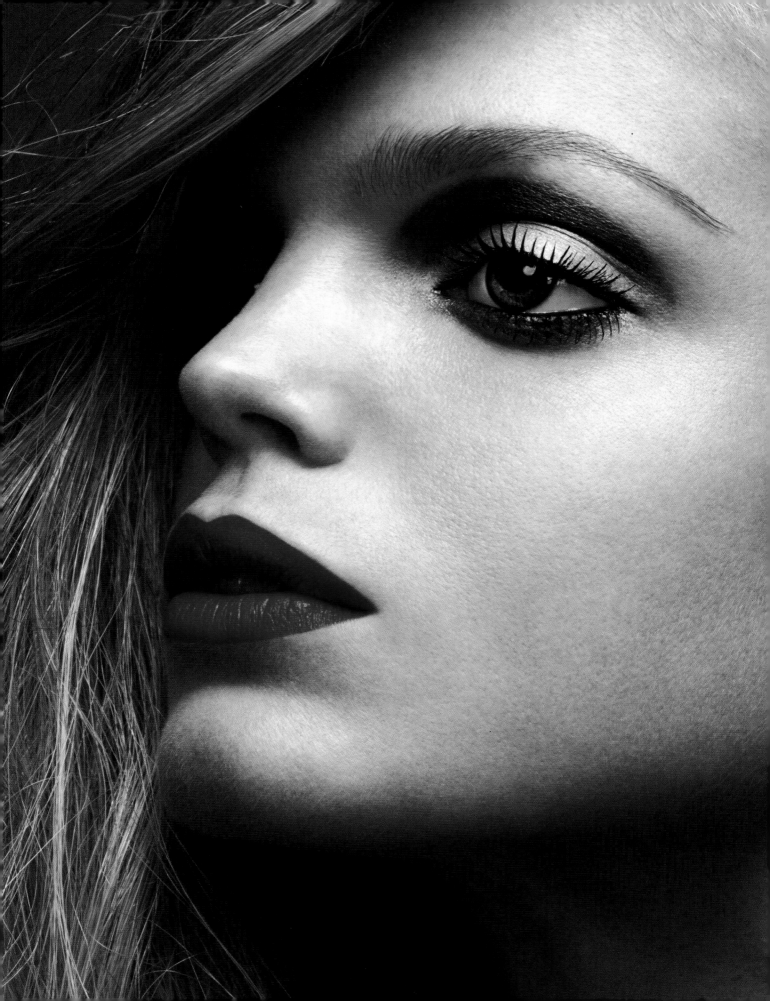

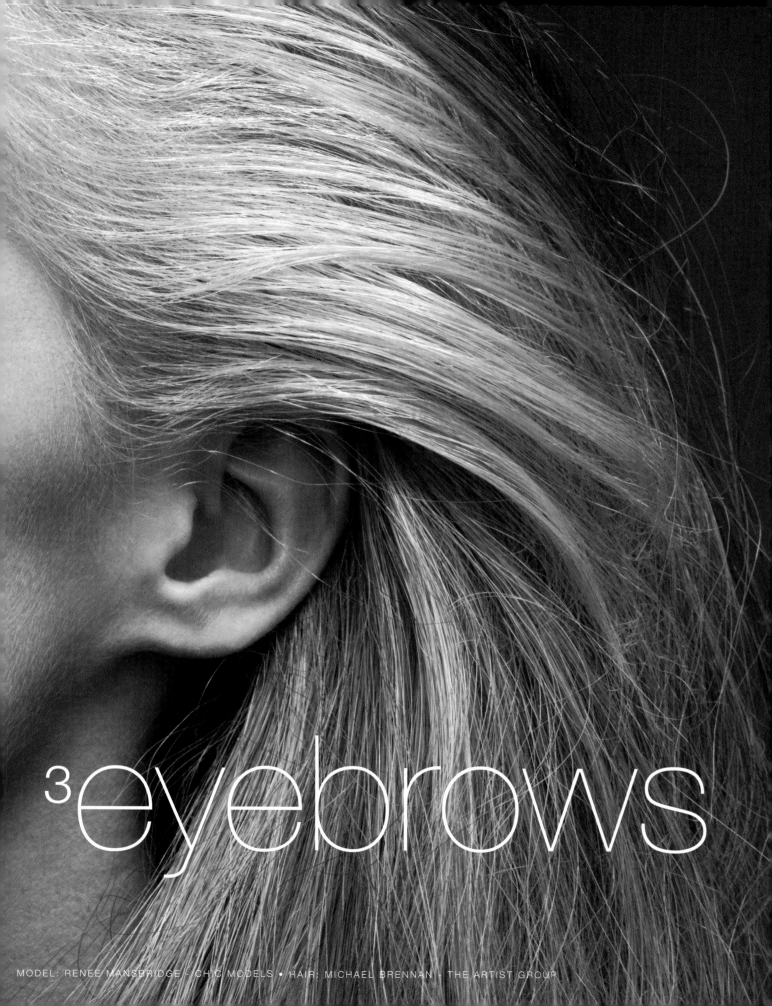

³eyebrows

When it comes to facial features, little has more power and impact than the shape of your brows. Get the shape right and you have an instant face-lift effect. Get it wrong and it can cause all sorts of problems. For instance, many women don't realise that their eyebrow shape can visually alter the look of their nose (for all the wrong reasons). What's more, the colour of your brows can either harden your features or take years off.

Great brows frame your eyes—they hold everything together and give your features definition and strength. As a makeup artist, when I'm shooting beauty for high-end fashion magazines, I always cast models based upon their brows.

If there is one section of this book I want you to take special notice of, it's this one. There's no point in doing glamorous or sexy eye makeup if you have eyebrows that look like caterpillars, slugs or tadpoles.

The number one 'crime' on my eyebrow offence list is over-plucked brows. Most women think that thin, highly arched brows lift the eye and make you look younger. However, they do the complete opposite. So let's start with the types of brows you should *not* have.

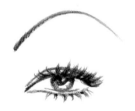

Type: Over-plucked. Hairs have been tweezed to oblivion, and there's barely a brow to be seen.
Effect: You've just aged yourself by ten years! Not to mention given yourself puffy-looking lids and a slight eye-droop.

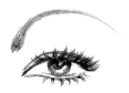

Type: Tadpole brows, aka commas.
Effect: Extremely unattractive. These brows do nothing for you and the question on every makeup artist's lips is: 'Why? Who did this to you? And have you looked at a clown lately?'

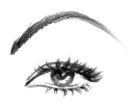

Type: The big 'M'. As in, semi-circle brows that look like they need a compass to navigate them.
Effect: First, these are the opposite of sophisticated (read: tarty). Second, they add five kilos instantly—this is the best way to add weight (in a bad way) to your face. Third, they make your nose look bigger. And fourth, they make your eyes look droopy.

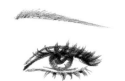

Type: The downhill.
Effect: Speaks for itself. Just look closer at this sketch: sad, sad eyes; hello, puffy eyelids. These brows do nothing but make you look haggard and tired.

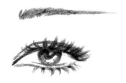

Type: The parting of the Red Sea.
Effect: Wide-set brows give you a blank expression and you look a little alien-ish. In terms of features, they throw the whole face out of balance, and they widen your nose like you would not believe.

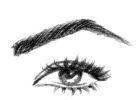

Type: The triangle.
Effect: These brows mean you're peaking too soon. By lifting the brow in the middle of the eye, you're causing a downhill puffy eyelid, and distorting your eye shape. It makes your eyebrows look like arrows pointing at the sky. This is a very hard look.

how to rehab your brows

If any of the above brows belong to you, then my advice is an urgent brow rehab! But if yours don't strictly fit in with these types of brows, how can you tell if your brows suit you? First, look at yourself closely in the mirror. Study your eyes and brows and then completely cover your brows with your index fingers. Look at your eyes again. Do they look better with or without your current brows? If the answer is 'without', this says that your brows are doing more harm than good to your look. Now, don't run for the wax pot! Book an appointment with a brow specialist (someone with good word-of-mouth reputation—ask your well-browed friends where they go), who will be able to design the perfect brow shape for you.

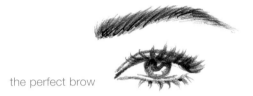

the perfect brow

How to achieve the perfect brows

Have you ever been told to start your eyebrows from an imaginary line upwards from your outer nostril or from the inner corner of your eye? In this scenario, if you have a wide nose or flared nostrils, you should start your brows closer to your eyeballs, with a huge gap in between. Right? Wrong!

As you can see from the photos opposite, a harsh arch in the wrong place can create a puffy eye and uneven brows are the right ingredients for a drooping or lopsided face. Likewise, a gap that is too big between a set of brows can actually make a nose look really big. That is why having the right brow shape is essential. The correct brow can make eyes look bigger, rectify unevenness, straighten your nose and make your face much more striking. In other words, the correct brow is important in making a beautiful face and therefore makeup.

The easiest way to achieve a foolproof brow is to follow a few small rules and three long lines.

1 Everyone has different-sized nostrils and noses, so your imaginary line must follow the natural line of the outer bridge of your nose. Got it? That is where your first brow hairs need to start! Then you can de-mono-brow all you like on the other side of this line.

2 Now, from that bridge line, draw another line that passes along the outer rim of your pupil and upwards. This is the highest point of any arch or height of the brow. This incline should smoothly follow the natural shape of your own brow. It's important to note that the arch isn't in the centre of the brow—it is very much off-centre, making the eye longer, sexier and with no 'surprised' look!

3 Finally, again, from the bridge line draw a line to the outer corner of your eye. This is where your brow should end.

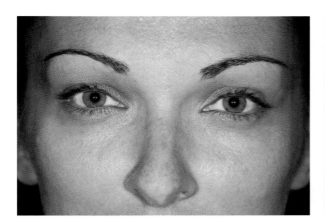

before (with over-plucked eyebrows)

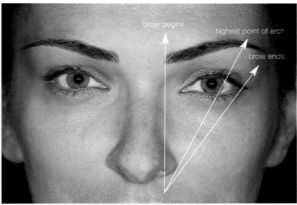

after (with the perfect eyebrows)

brow lightening

DO NOT TRY THIS AT HOME. Brow lightening must only be done by a fully qualified hairdresser because it's not as easy as it looks, and as you are working very close to the eye, you can cause some damage if you don't do it properly. You know how difficult it can be to colour the hair on your head; well, the same qualifications are needed to bleach brows (that's why hardly any makeup artists do it).

So why lighten? Because lightening the brows can be one of the most 'softening' techniques you can do. It's great when you change your hair colour—for example, if you go from being a blonde to a redhead, by colouring your brows a soft chestnut it makes your new hair colour look more natural, and it will soften your overall look. What's more, bleaching your brows has a softening effect on the hair itself, which is fantastic if you have brow hair like barbed wire.

If you want to lighten your brows but are a little scared about how they may end up looking, you can take a sneak preview by using brow mascaras (or hair mascaras—they were horrible on the hair to which they were supposed to add highlights, so due to bad sales they are hard to find, but they are fantastic on the brows). Just comb the colour mascara on and see what it looks like.

You can also darken your brows. As brow hairs fall out in cycles every six to eight weeks, any colour change is never permanent.

So to sum up, don't try it at home, and test brow-colour changes by using brow mascaras. And remember, it's only hair, and if you don't like it you can colour it back.

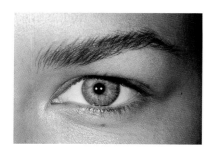

before lightening

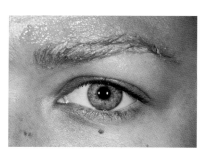

during lightening

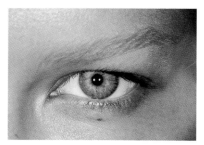

after lightening

brow tips

1 Your brows must suit you! If they don't, get them shaped by a professional.

2 Trim any extra-long hairs on your brows, but ideally, this would be done by your brow expert (even your hairdresser can come in handy for this one).

3 Always check brows from the side—use a second mirror to see your profile view.

4 Match your brow pencil to your brow hair colour, not your desired hair colour, as the difference would be too obvious.

5 If you lighten your hair colour on your head, then consider lightening your brows.

6 Buy brow mascaras—my favourite tool in this area. They are great for temporarily lightening or darkening the brow, as they have a gel formula which holds them into place. Brow mascara comes in many colours; if you're a redhead, you can buy one that matches your head hair colour, to tonally tie everything together.

7 Don't wax your brows on the day of an important event, because wax removes a light layer of skin and makes it impossible for foundation and eye shadow to adhere.

4false

eyelashes

false lashes are like shoes—they either fit or they don't! If they don't fit correctly, they are uncomfortable, they can fall off or, worse, they will look fake when you don't want them to.

As a makeup artist, I use some sort of false lash in nearly every makeup I do. My two favourite things in makeup are mascara (as important as the air we breathe) and false lashes. If I don't have lashes in my kit, I go into a complete panic and I'll send assistants running for miles. I have even been caught cutting tiny hairs from models' heads (without them noticing) and sticking them on—now, that's desperation!

Most women don't realise that lashes, when applied by professionals, are measured to fit your exact lash line. This involves measuring the lash line and comparing it with the length of the false lash, and if it's too long or too short either the false lash has to be cut, or single lashes need to be added. You can do this yourself. Remember that 80 per cent of lashes will fit all eye shapes, but if the ones you buy are too long, then all you need to do is cut them.

I have found that in most cases a full lash is not required. For me, the sexiest look is when single lashes or just one-quarter is used on the outer lash line; this gives a winged effect and lifts the eyes instantly.

You can reuse false lashes (I don't because of hygiene). If you're using them for your eyes only, just soak them in warm water for 5 minutes to remove the glue before reusing.

As with anything there are do's and don'ts, so before you launch yourself into applying false lashes take note of the following.

Don't

- overuse glue, as it will not dry and can go into your eyes
- apply the lash if the glue is too wet; just squeeze a tiny amount onto the back of your hand and wait for it to get a little tacky, then apply it to the back of the false lash—not your lash line
- trim the false lash after you have applied it; you can cut your own lashes (I guarantee it!)—this is strictly for professionals only
- use lashes that are too heavy for your natural lashes to hold, as they drag your lash line down
- apply lashes too far out on your lash line if you have rounded eyes as they will drag your lash line down (see illustrations opposite).

Do

- curl your own lashes before applying falsies; if you attempt it afterwards, you can rip them off
- check the base of the lash; for example, if the lash (being a full lash) has a black line at its base, remember it will give you the look of an eyeliner, which you may or may not want
- paint the base after application if it is white (use liquid liner).

applying false eyelashes

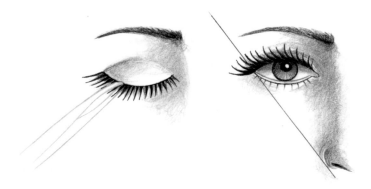

This illustration (above) clearly demonstrates how NOT to apply a false lash. As you can see, if you are looking down and apply the lash all the way to the end of your natural lash line, when you look up the false lash will drag down, causing the eye to droop. Also, it can cause a nasty shadow under the eye.

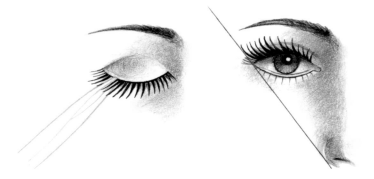

This is the correct way to apply false lashes. Notice that the lash has been moved inwards about half a centimetre. This ensures that when you look straight ahead, your lashes follow that beautiful line that gives your eyes a lift (from the corner of the nose to the corner of your eye). This instantly makes you look YOUNGER. The same applies with a single lash: always start approximately half a centimetre inwards. This rule rarely applies for Asian eyes because the eyelid is straighter and you don't have the issue of the lash drooping on the ends.

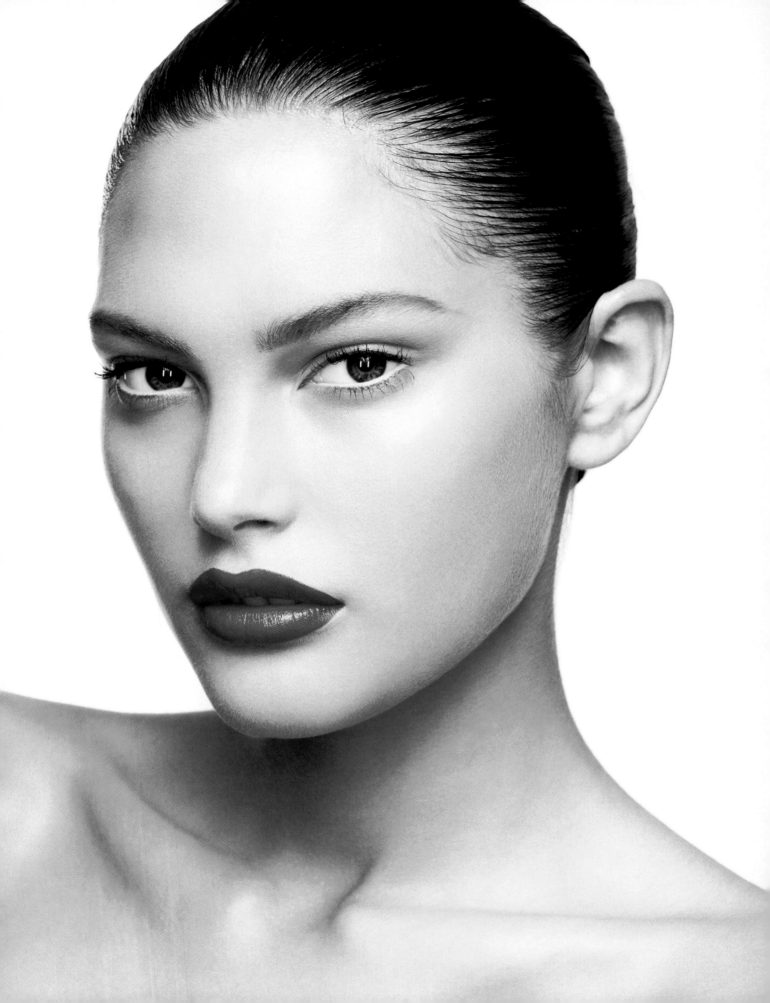

the power of lashes

I have used the next few pages to show you that false lashes have the power to dramatically change the way your eyes look. You can completely alter your eye makeup with just a lash. There are many different types of false lashes on the market. In fact, there are so many, no one would blame you for feeling confused and overwhelmed. So, over the next six pages, I show you three of the many possibilities you can achieve with false lashes.

In the first shot opposite, Catherine McNeil is not wearing false lashes. I have only applied a light layer of mascara to her eyes, as well as foundation and lipstick. Her makeup doesn't change over the following pages, only her lashes do. And you can see the difference in each shot.

Eyelash glue

Most eyelashes are sold with a complementary lash glue. But I would recommend that you buy a tube of professional eyelash glue, that is sold separately, from any quality makeup store, because these complementary glues don't adhere very well. In the false lash glue family, there are three types:

- **Standard glue**, which is white in colour and dries clear.
- **Waterproof and higher strength**, also white in colour and dries clear. I would recommend this glue for the heavy lash that needs more support.
- **Black eyelash glue**. I definitely recommend this when using a black liquid eyeliner or a black smoky eye shadow as it will be undetectable, unlike the clear-drying glue which you might be able to see with black.

35

natural lashes

On Catherine's first shot, I have applied a feathery single-strip lash. I call this the J.Lo lash, as she's known for it. With this lash, you can apply mascara either before or after you place it on your eyes. Just remember, the glue must be dry if you're applying mascara afterwards, because the slightest tension can pull the lash off.

These lashes are great for

- all eye shapes
- lifting the eyes
- opening the eye more; a tip here—apply mascara to the bottom lash as well (in this shot, I have applied mascara on top of the false lash and a subtle amount to the bottom lashes).

General tip

Whenever I'm doing shows and all the models are having the same makeup look using false lashes, even though the makeup is to look the same I find myself using completely different lashes to achieve this because of the different eye shapes. So my point is, remember that lashes are like shoes— you need to fit them; some will be too long, short, wide or heavy. A great way to check you have used the right ones is to look straight up, hold a mirror underneath and check that the false lash blends with yours, and that there are no gaps.

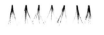

knot free flare long black

Lashes used here

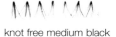

flare under black

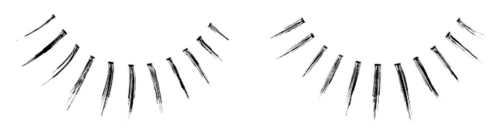

knot free medium black

36

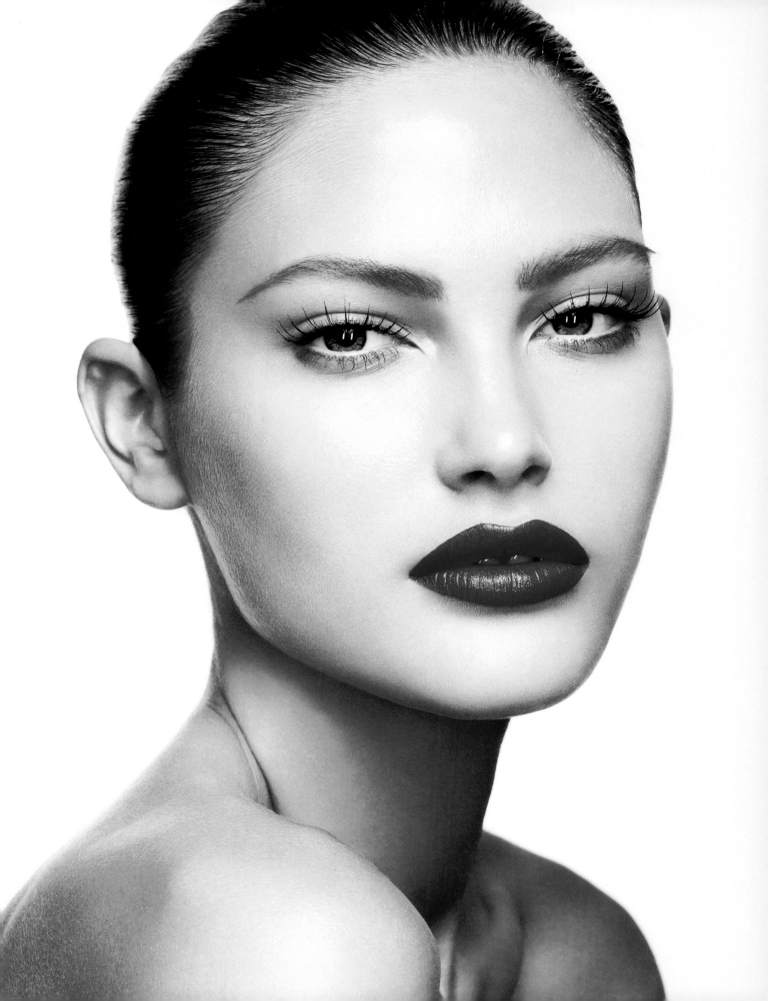

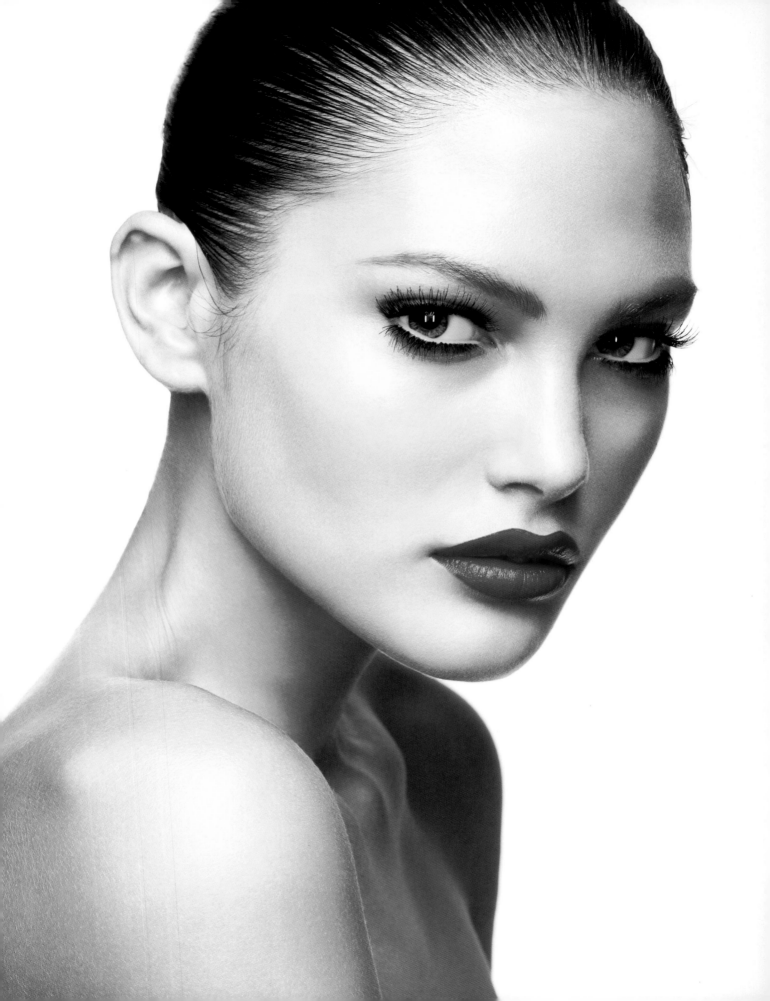

lux lashes

I call this look the 'eye-opener'. The best way to enlarge your eyes is to apply lashes to both top and bottom. Yes, I admit it's not easy to do, so let me take you through it step by step and give you great tips.

I like to apply all the single bottom lashes first (and after applying mascara). Why? Because when we blink, the lashes have a habit of sticking themselves to the top lash (very annoying and time-consuming).

There are two ways of applying bottom lashes: you either apply the glue 'under' the false lash then stick the lashes 'on top' of your natural lash, or you apply the glue 'on top' of the false lash then apply it 'under' your natural lash. A little confusing, I know, but you need to give this one a few goes to get it right.

Wait until all the lash glue has completely dried before you apply the top lashes or they will stick together. You can tell when the glue has dried because it goes clear (use white glue not black on the bottom lash).

Once you have achieved the bottom lash (and haven't ripped your hair out), the top is easy. Add a little glue to each individual lash, then apply one by one (as I have used individual lashes).

General tips

When using single top lashes, apply them mostly to the outer corners as this lifts the eyes and gives them a sexy look.

You can use full-strip lashes underneath—just make sure they are not too long or too wide. There are so many on the market, you just need to find the best fit.

Lashes used here

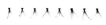

flare under black

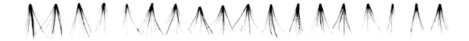

39

high-impact lashes

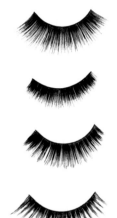

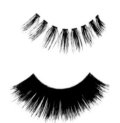

This one speaks for itself. I have applied a heavy-strip lash; note that I haven't changed her makeup at all. Isn't it amazing what a lash can do? Apply mascara before putting on the lash, and keep the mascara to the top lash only, because it can start to look a little draggy!

These lashes are great for

- anyone who's game to wear them
- larger sized eyes
- Asian eyes.

These are not recommended for

- very rounded eyes
- small eyes
- eyes with few natural lashes (remember the false lashes need support).

General tip

Because this lash is extremely heavy, it needs support, so don't use one this thick if you have very few of your own lashes (see options on the left), because it will just keep dropping. And in most cases, you have to hold the lash up to your lash line and make sure the strip is not too long. Often, I will cut a few millimetres off the longest end of the false lash so it fits well, and apply extra glue especially on the ends.

Lashes used here

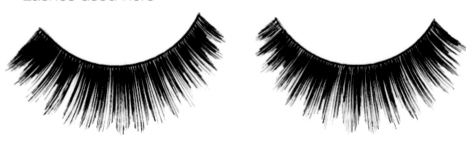

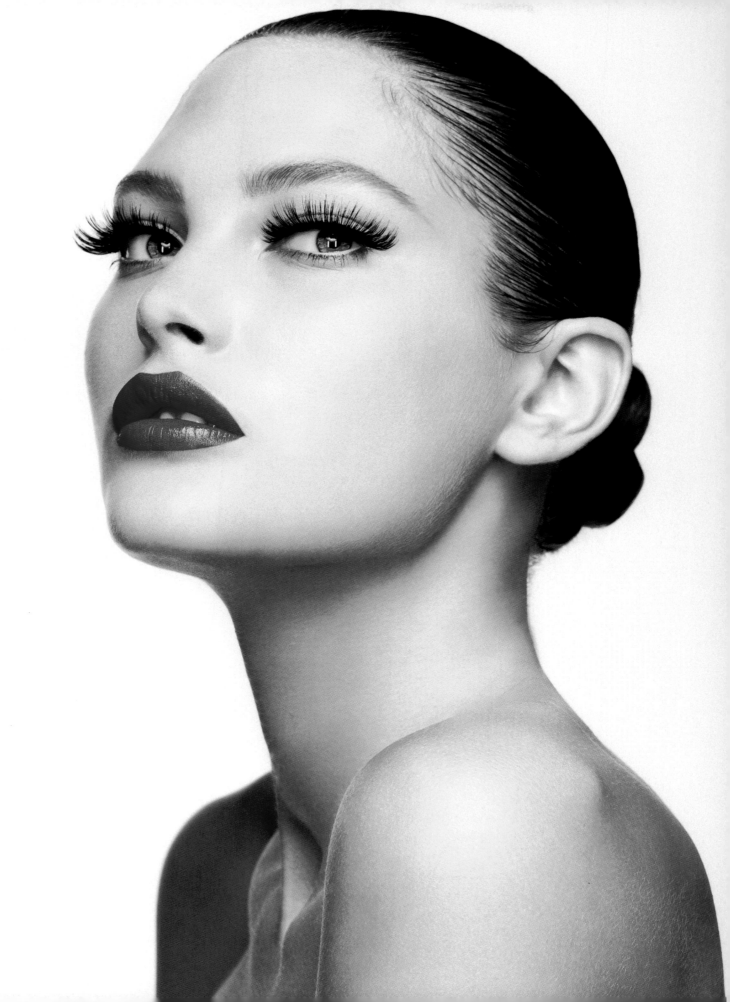

⁵eye colour

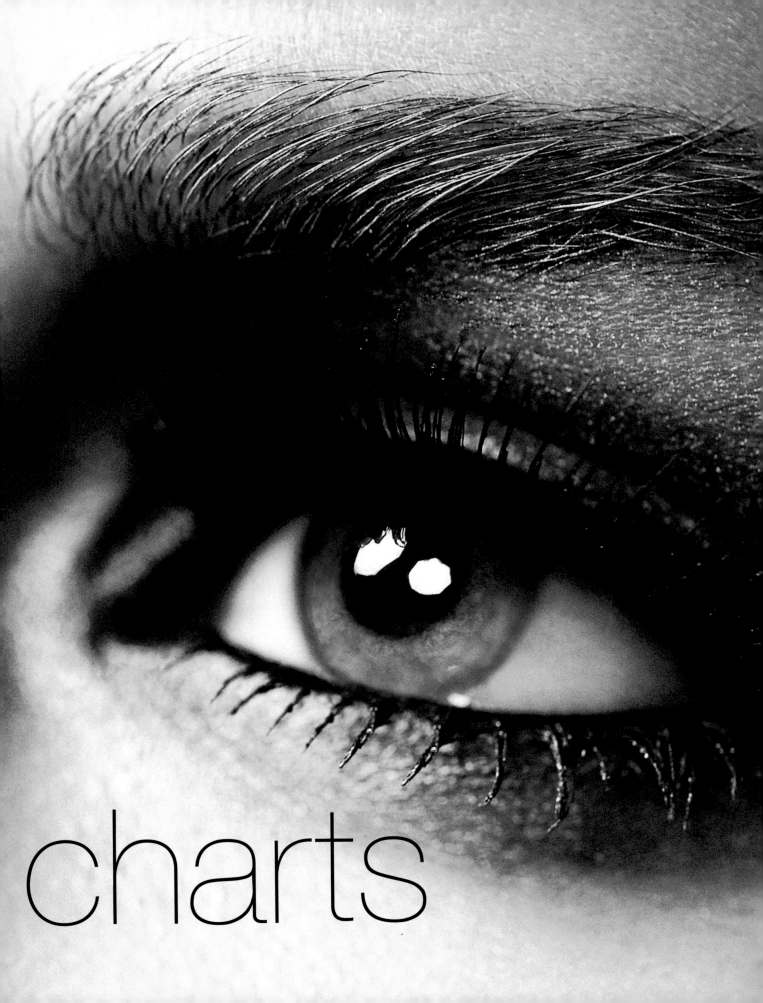

charts

o you know the number one question I get asked? 'What colour suits me?' (Actually, the number one question I get asked is 'Will you do the makeup for my wedding?' but 'What colour suits me?' is certainly a close second.) And although it's a great question (the colour one, not the wedding one), it's also a question which is very difficult to answer.

Why? Because half the time, the women asking me have got the wrong hair colour, the wrong-coloured clothing and the wrong accessories. And they are hoping that the 'right' lipstick will somehow magically pull the whole ensemble together.

Now, I am a makeup artist not a magician, and there is only so much that makeup can achieve. But what I will say is this: I believe wearing the wrong colour around your eyes is worse than wearing the wrong-coloured shirt (although I did see some shirts in Hawaii that nearly caused me to revise my opinion). And I dare say that if you get your makeup colours right, you can get away with wearing a coloured top that may not technically be one of your best or most flattering shades.

So because I take this topic very seriously, I consulted an expert in colour science. Bronwyn Fraser knows more about colour and the science of colour than anyone else I know, with years of experience working within the hair, beauty and fashion industries and also as a personal stylist. So you can trust that the following text is scientifically sound. (You can check out Bronwyn's website www.styleestablishment.com.au)

'There are no rules when it comes to fashion' … how often do we hear that quote? This is certainly true to an extent, as any makeup artist or fashion stylist will tell you, and the 'rules' are often broken to create a wow-factor or dramatic visual effect for magazine shoots or fashion shows. When it comes to selecting clothes, makeup, accessories or basically anything worn above the waist, the very first checkpoint for me is always colour, before cut, fit, style, fabric or anything else! Get the colour right and you are more than halfway there.

There are individual colours or colour families we can all wear to enhance and harmonise our natural colouring and emphasise our number one feature—our EYES! Always remember, your eyes are the first feature anyone sees when they look at your face, followed by your lips. To understand some easy colour basics when choosing your eye colours, refer to the eye colour charts in the following pages.

Highlighters/enhancers

These shades will really open up your eyes. You won't always find this written on the package but basically they are colours that highlight or reflect your own natural eye colour—don't worry we have worked that out for you in the colour charts.

Intensifiers/poppers

These colours, on an artist's colour wheel, are made of predominantly the opposite pigments to your own eyes, and therefore provide maximum contrast value to really brighten and illuminate your natural eye colour.

Neutrals

These are shades which are considered 'neutral' as they are made of varying combinations of the three primary colours, blue, red and yellow. There are warmer browns containing more yellow pigments that are suited to warmer brown, green and hazel eyes, and cooler browns containing more blue pigments best suited to deep brown, blue, cool green and cool hazel eyes, yet all do contain a combination of the three primary colours in their mix. Shades of brown eye shadow are universal and can be worn by anyone, any time, for a natural or sophisticated look depending on how it is applied.

Metallics

These high-shine reflective shades can be warm, cool or neutral and a little goes a long way! Metallic shades will draw maximum attention to wherever they are applied (many highlighters are metallic), so if your skin is less than perfect, be aware as metallics will highlight any flaws or fine lines. Used all over, they will give a beautiful, fresh sheen for both daytime and evening.

Accents

These are deep, vivid or bright colours used on either the upper or lower eye areas and are best applied in minimal quantities, such as a fine line very close to the lash line or a corner accent on either the inner and/or outer corners, for that extra impact. Think of these as 'accessory' shades, just like a great pair of shoes, handbag or earrings to complete a look.

blue eyes

Select your eye tone

ALL BLUE EYES

Eye shadows

WARM BLUES

Best shadow for all warm
blue-coloured eyes

COOL BLUES

Best shadow for all cool
blue-coloured eyes

ALL BLUES

Shades to intensify and make
all blue eyes 'pop'

Eye-shadow pigments to highlight and enhance

ALL BLUE EYES

Metallics

Enhancers

Eyeliners

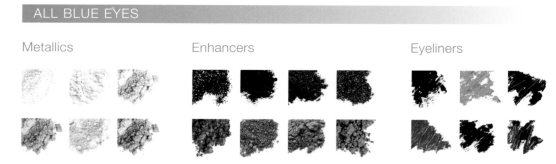

green eyes

Select your eye tone

ALL GREEN EYES

Eye shadows

WARM GREENS
Best shadow for all warm green-coloured eyes

COOL GREENS
Best shadow for all cool green-coloured eyes

ALL GREENS
Shades to intensify and make all green eyes 'pop'

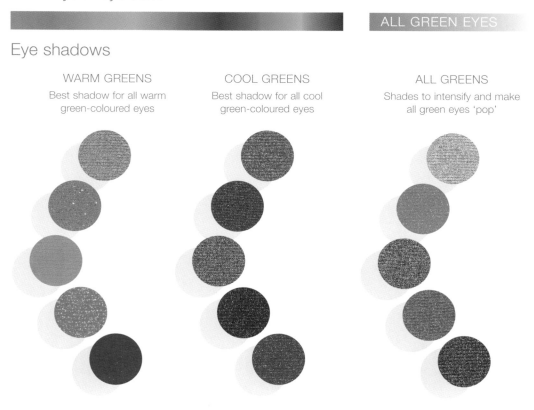

Eye-shadow pigments to highlight and enhance

ALL GREEN EYES

Metallics

Enhancers

Eyeliners

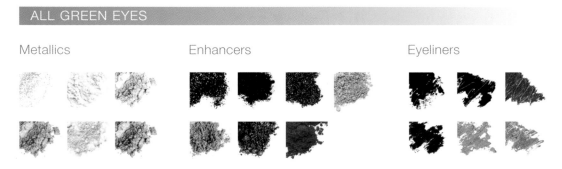

brown eyes

Select your eye tone

ALL BROWN EYES

Eye shadows

WARM BROWNS
Best shadow for all warm
brown-coloured eyes

COOL BROWNS
Best shadow for all cool
brown-coloured eyes

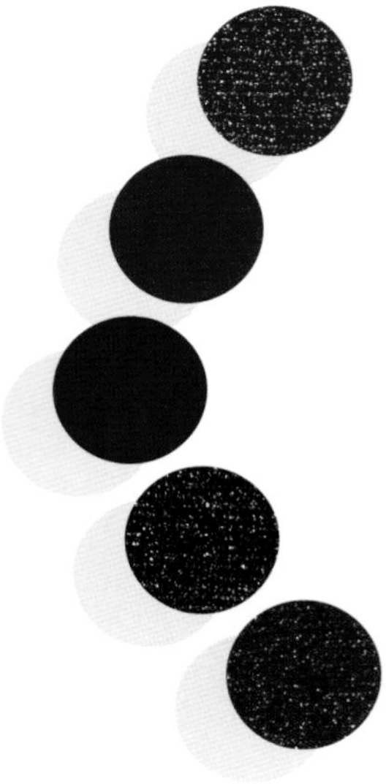

ALL BROWNS
Shades to intensify and make
all brown eyes 'pop'

Eye-shadow pigments to highlight and enhance

ALL BROWN EYES

Metallics

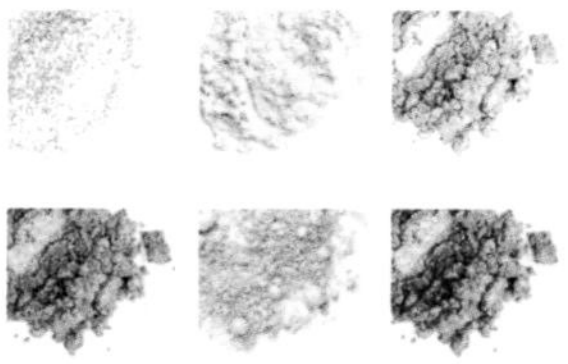

Enhancers

Eyeliners

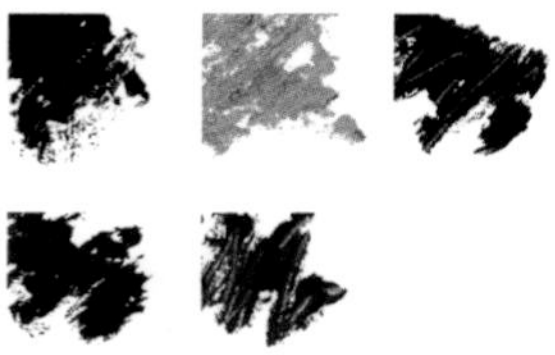

hazel eyes

Select your eye tone

Eye shadows

TRUE HAZELS
Best shadow for all
green/hazel-coloured eyes

GOLDS
Best shadow for all warm/golden
hazel-coloured eyes

ALL HAZELS
Shades to intensify and make
all hazel eyes 'pop'

Eye-shadow pigments to highlight and enhance

ALL HAZEL EYES

Metallics

Enhancers

Eyeliners

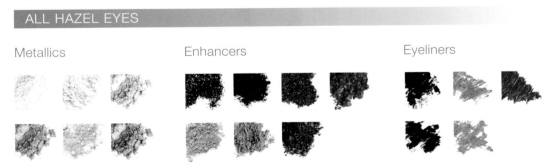

neutrals

These are considered neutral shades and can be worn by all eye colours, any time.

Eye shadows for all eye colours

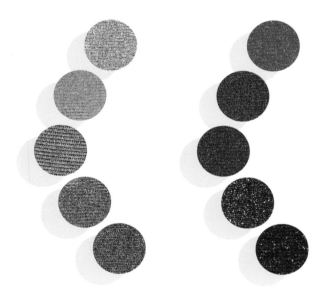

Eye-shadow pigments to highlight and enhance

ALL EYES

Metallics

Enhancers

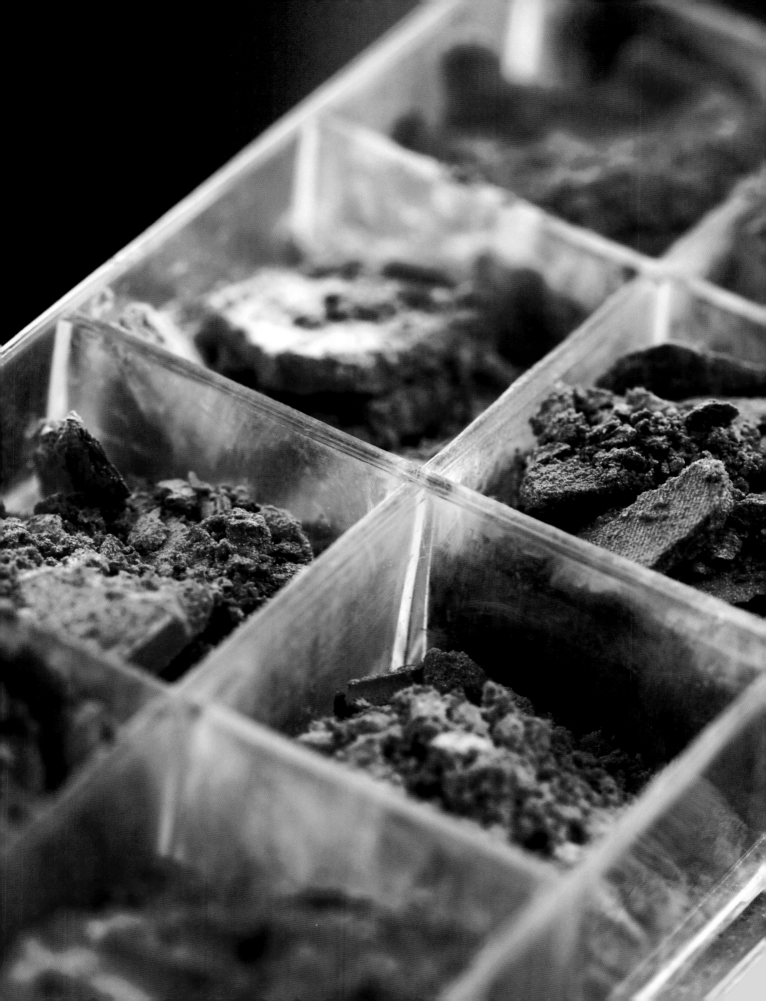

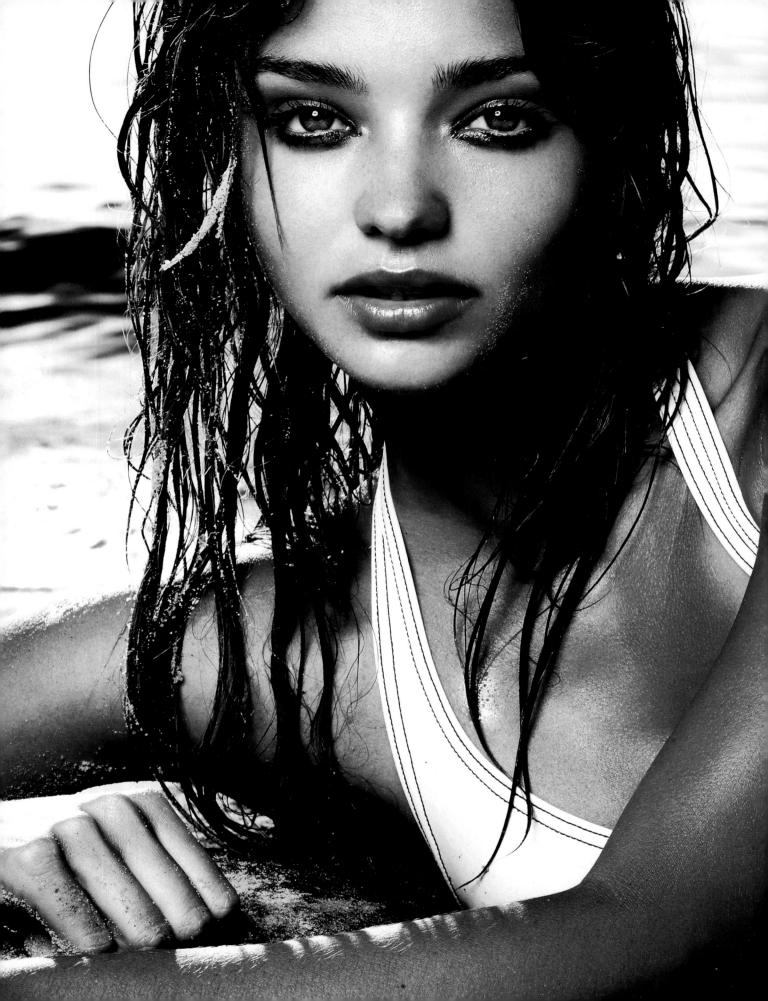

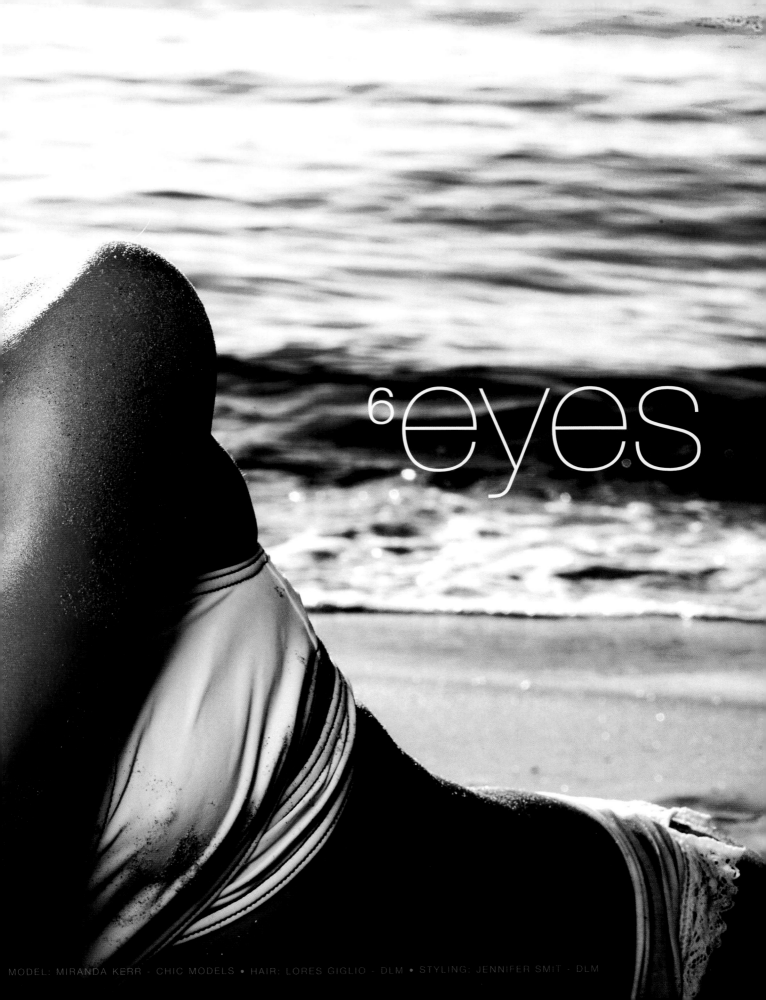

⁶eyes

You've probably noticed that the order of things in this book is slightly unusual compared with other makeup books. Most makeup books will tell you how to do the foundation first, and then how to conceal before you begin your eye makeup. But my philosophy is different. I've given you the Eyes chapter before the rest. Why? Because the eyes are the most powerful feature in the face, and I believe they should be done first.

Whether you have large, small, round, almond-shaped or Asian eyes, they are the first thing anyone notices. So how you tackle them, in a makeup sense, is crucial. The eyes are the key to successful makeup. They mirror all your efforts in trying to achieve a certain look. But more than that, they affect everything, including the overall shape of your face. If you get the eyes right, you've pretty much nailed it.

I do the eyes first for two main reasons. First, it avoids that nasty little thing known as 'fallout'. Fallout is that annoying eye shadow that continually drops on your cheeks, usually after you have applied your foundation, which you constantly have to wipe off. It wastes a lot of time and ruins your foundation. (Sorbolene cream is terrific for gently removing fallout.)

Second, I find that most women only allocate minimal time to do their makeup in the mornings, and yet they spend most of this time doing foundation! It doesn't make sense to put all your energy and effort into doing what's easy—the foundation—when you should be concentrating on what takes the longest and is the most intricate—your eyes. You can always do your foundation in the car on the way to work (I certainly do), on the train (most women will just think you're applying sunscreen anyway), or in the bathroom at work just before you enter the office.

If you do your eyes first, and you don't like how they look when you're done, then you can simply wipe it off and start again WITHOUT having to redo your base. But before you do any eye makeup, YOU MUST PREP YOUR EYES. Remember, your eyelids are one of the oiliest parts of your face, so please don't apply more oil to them. I've given you step-by-step instructions on how to prep your eyes in the Skin Prepping chapter (see page 21) so please use them!

How to achieve great eye makeup

Eye makeup is about knowing what you have, and knowing how to enhance it. Take a close look at your eyes and determine:

- what colour are they?
- what shape are they?
- what don't you like about your eyes?

The eye colour charts I've given you in this book (see pages 46–50) will help you work out which colours best suit your eyes. There's an amazing variety of eye shadows, pencils, mascaras, false eyelashes, etc., all designed to make you look fantastic. Keep on referring to the colour charts, especially as you consider new looks and colours, either at the makeup counter or as you read the book, and don't be afraid to experiment. In the case of the eyes, practice makes perfect.

Throughout this chapter, I talk about creating a wash over the eyelids. A wash is a primary colour, representing the tone you're going to use. If you're going to create eye makeup with a blue intensity, for example, you would begin with a wash of blue. It's purely a base of colour. Everything else is for the shape. A wash:

- can be soft or intense
- refers to the application, and is not a pastel beginning
- can be either dry or wet
- can be applied either to the middle lid or over the whole eyelid area (this is explained in every step-by-step in the following pages).

You'll also notice that I use metallic colours in this chapter. When using metallic colours on the lower lash line of the eyes, it's crucial to keep them very close to the lash line. If you let metallic colours drop too low, it will look like you haven't slept in weeks, it will magnify any fine lines and make them look worse, and will make you look like an old member of the Spice Girls. To top things off, it can also have a scaling effect. ALL TO BE AVOIDED.

Eye shape

The most common problem with eye shape is that often women don't know what to do to minimise or enhance a certain shape. Whatever your eye shape, my golden rule is to NEVER DO THINGS IN HALF on the eye. You should always extend lines and shadows either one-third or two-thirds of the way. If you do anything halfway across, it cuts the eye in half and makes it look distorted.

So let's address the biggest problems with shape:

If you have small eyes

You can make them look larger. The best trick in the book is to curl your lashes (apply mascara, of course), and apply creamy white pencil (not waterproof) to the inner rim. This creates an illusion of larger eyes. If you feel confident, adding single false lashes to the top outer lash line will also enlarge the eyes (see the False Eyelashes chapter, page 30). Check out the Asian Eyes chapter (page 120) for even more tips.

If you have very large, rounded or protruding eyes

Never use hard-edged eyeliner, either above or below; a smudged liner is the only type allowed. Hard-edged liner results in framing the eye and bringing attention to the roundness. I love to make this eye shape more cat-like by applying dark pencil to the inner rim of the eye; this helps to shrink the eye shape. Keep all dark colours to the outer third corner of the eye, and if you want to create a smoky effect don't follow the natural shape of the eye; the outline should be more of a square shape—the trick is to make the eye shadow into a more rectangular shape—i.e. don't follow the natural roundness of the eye—and to extend the outer corner of the eye. Don't highlight the middle of the eyelid, and only apply mascara to the top lashes.

If you have heavy eyelids

Whatever colour you choose as your eye shadow, use it in the inner corners (top and bottom) of your eyes. This way, if your eyes are open, you can still see the colour on your lids (i.e. it won't get covered by the heavy lid). Eyebrow shape is essential; anything too arched will accentuate heavy lids, so you want a straighter brow shape with a slight arch. No frosty eye shadow allowed for heavy eyelids (see *Kath & Kim* for reference)! However, using a matt contouring shade on the lids is a great way of giving the illusion of a deeper set socket (see the Contouring chapter on page 158).

If you have close-set eyes

The best tip is to use highlighter in the inner corners. Any darkening or shading or smoking is to be restricted to the outer corner of the eye—this includes keeping the false eyelashes on the outer corner. So the basic rule is that everything that is light or highlighting or metallic goes on the inner part of the eye and anything dark or smoky goes on the outer part of the eye, to 'wing' it out. If you darken the eye the whole way across, you actually make the problem more obvious.

If you have very small eyelashes

The solution is easy—use false lashes! I've given you a whole chapter on this, and I've used them in almost every step-by-step in this chapter, so there's no excuse!

Smoky eyes

One of my favourites! Most people probably think this is too harsh or over the top for the average woman, or that it's too difficult to achieve. But smoky eyes don't have to be harsh; they can be subtle and sexy yet keep the eyes open and fresh and still give that fantastic impact.

My tips for smoky eyes:
- Lining the inner eye with a creamy white pencil will open up the eyes.
- Lining the eyes with black gives you a cat-like effect.
- You can't go past deep violet tones for smoky eyes, especially when you're wearing black.
- There is no eye shape that is not suited to smoky eyes.
- If you want to add a little more colour, just hit the inner corner of your eyelids with a bright lavender, gold or blue. Metallic colours are best.
- Smoky eyes are fantastic for women with small lips; focusing on the eyes takes the attention off the lips.
- If done properly, smoky eyes don't have to be touched up after the initial application.
- Remember, they don't have to be black and dark. You can achieve smoky eyes with bronzed colours, a jewelled effect, and even shades of green.

In the following pages, I will show you the unedited 'real deal' when applying makeup. NONE of the step-by-steps have been retouched. I will show you ways of creating strong, glamorous, sexy eyes.

Remember, before you begin:
- Prep your eyes first.
- Oil and heavy eye creams will destroy eye makeup.
- Lightly powder the eyes to blend your eye shadow.
- Sorbolene cream is a great tool for gently removing fallout under the eye.

bronzed eyes

Because you're applying the eye shadow wet, you must not look up for at least 30 seconds, as it will cause the makeup to crease.

Using an antique gold as opposed to a yellow gold looks more elegant.

Use powder on the eyelid to blend the rest of the eye shadow.

Once your eye is complete, take the same gold you used on the lid and apply to the inner corner of the eye and to the cupid's bow of your lips.

For a more dramatic look, apply single/individual false lashes to the outer corners of the upper lash line.

The gold and bronze colour palettes look amazing on blue eyes.

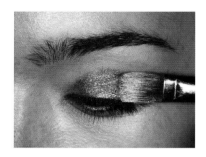

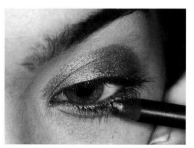

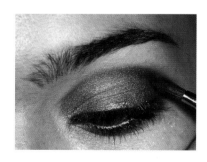

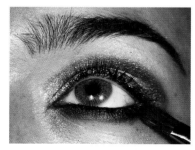

1 Prep the eyelid, making sure it is well powdered all around; this will help you to blend eye shadows better. Using a wet medium brush, apply antique gold eye shadow to the entire eyelid. Wetting the brush will minimise fallout and intensify the gold.

2 Overload the inner rim of the eye with an antique gold eye pencil—don't be afraid to load it up. Make sure the pencil you use is not waterproof. Eye pencil used in the inner rim disappears quickly due to blinking, etc., so ensure constant reapplication for a lasting look.

3 Using a smaller brush, finely apply a rusty brown eye shadow along the socket line. If you find this isn't blending, then go back to the first step and powder well. Intensify the brown shadow in the outer corner of the eye.

4 Apply the same rusty brown eye colour all the way along the lower lash line. Curl lashes using a curler, and apply lots of jet-black mascara to both top and bottom lashes.

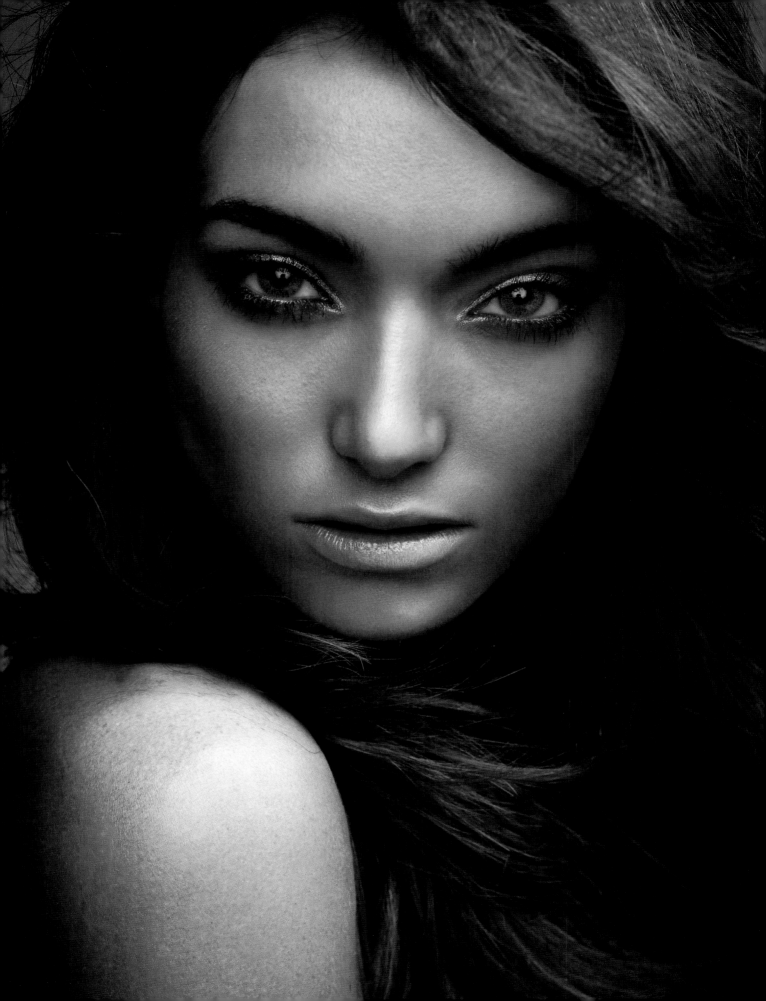

lavender eyes

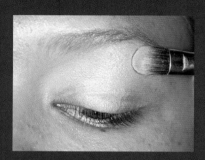

1 Using a pure white pencil, apply heavily to the inner eye rim. (Note: you will have to apply this again at the end.) Using a pearlised (has a pearl reflection) gold eye shadow, apply to the middle of the eyelid, then carry it right up to the brow bone.

TIPS

This eye shadow is not recommended for puffy eyelids, however, if you are using for puffy lids don't carry it all the way up to the brow bone. Instead, stop just above the lid.

If you have blonde lashes, wear brown mascara.

If you don't want such a heavy-lashed effect, apply a thick coating of brown mascara without using the false eyelashes.

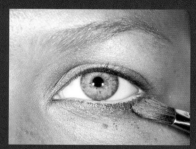

2 Apply a lavender eye shadow from the inner corner of the eye socket, blending up to the eyebrow and along the lower lash line. Make sure you keep the lid golden and don't carry the lavender too far across the upper lid.

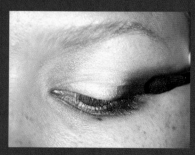

3 Smudge a little black kohl pencil into the top outer corner of the eye. Load up a small brush with dark violet eye shadow and blend it up and out as shown. Notice the eye is never closed—this gives you a smoother finish and stops the eye shadow from creasing.

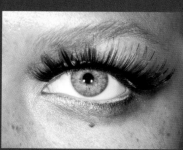

4 Because gold and lavender are such soft colours, I have strengthened the look by using full, strong, brown (not black) false eyelashes. Notice the little bit of white along the lash line. It's eyelash glue that will dry in 5 minutes (it's white when it's wet, clear when dry).

MODEL: LARA BINGLE • HAIR: KAREN HOPWOOD - DLM

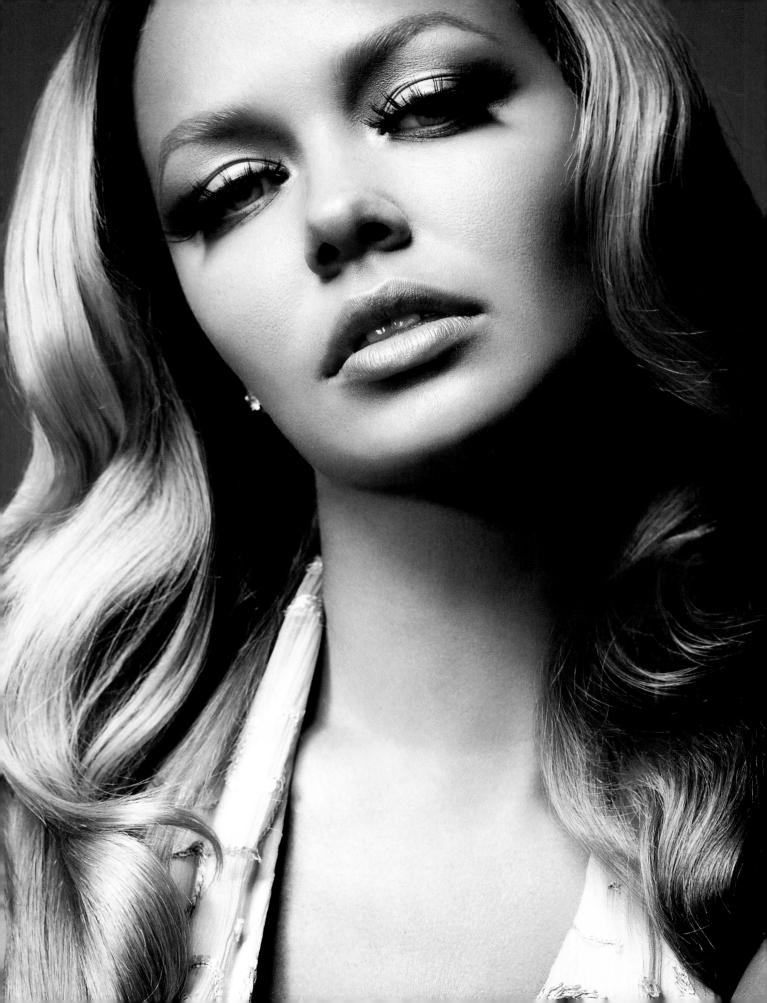

jewelled eyes

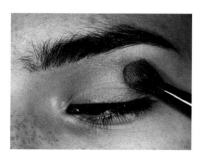

1 Prep the eyelid by making sure it is powdered well. Using a large brush, apply a light wash of soft coral eye shadow along the eye socket, blending up to the brow bone.

TIPS

This look is recommended for light olive to darker-toned skin.

This makeup looks best with strong top false lashes: it frames the eye.

For a cat-like eye effect, add mascara to the top lash line only. Only use black. Then finish off by using a soft gold highlighter under the brow.

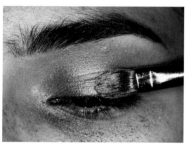

2 Using a large brush, cover the whole eyelid with an intense violet pigment, stopping just under the brow bone. Don't worry at this point about fallout— you can clean it up later. You can wet the brush to intensify the colour quickly.

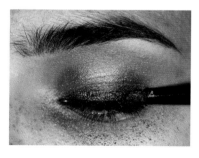

3 Using a smaller brush, intensify the lash line by applying a deeper shade of purple along the upper eyelid. You can also use a deep violet pencil or cream eyeliner to do this.

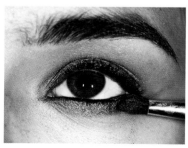

4 Clean up the drops of shadow that have fallen under the eye. Lightly base and powder under the eye (using a light dust of translucent powder for blending purposes). Then finish by applying an aqua-green pencil to the inner eye rim and shadow to the lower lash line, then mascara to the top and bottom lashes.

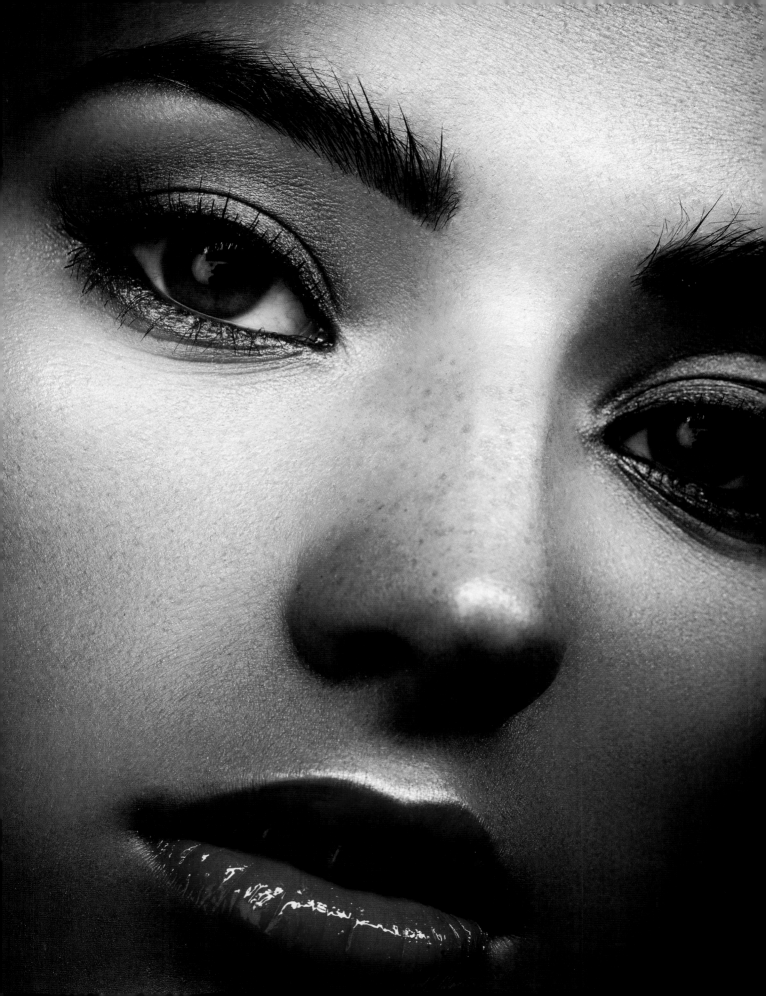

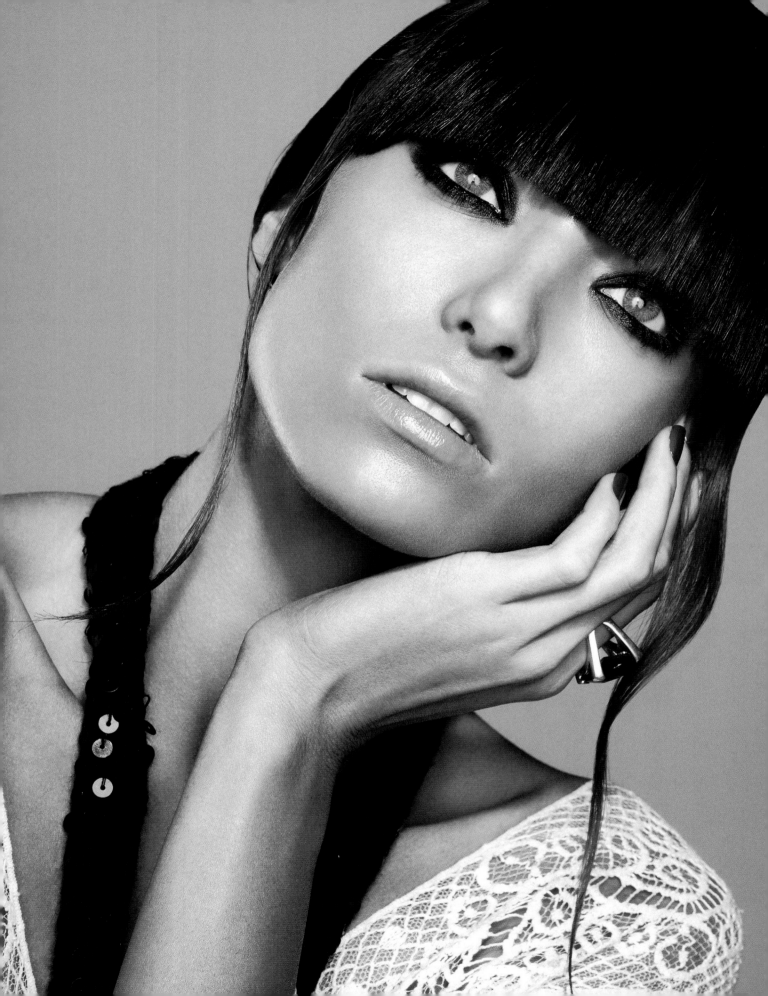

rock chick eyes

1 Apply an intense black kohl pencil or cream eyeliner to the inner rim and cover the entire eyelid; smudge with your finger. When lining the lower outer corner of the eye, smudge the pencil into and just below the lash line. The colour must be jet-black, otherwise it'll look dirty.

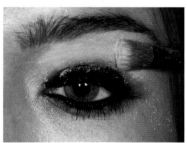

2 Using translucent powder that matches your skin tone, apply to the rest of the eye socket up to the brow bone. This will make the next stage much easier to blend.

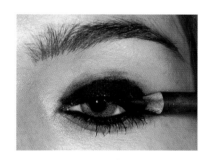

3 Dab some Sorbolene cream under the eye to make removing any dropped shadow easier (and avoid rubbing the skin). Using a small brush, apply dark metallic midnight-blue pigment to blend the black and lift the shape higher to just under the brow bone.

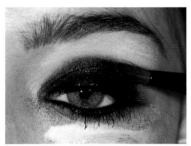

4 Apply the blue metallic pigment to the inner corner of the eye and underneath the lower lash line. Finish by applying lots of black mascara to the top and bottom lashes.

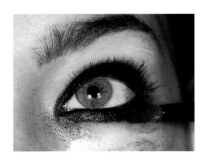

TIPS

Black fallout is hard to remove, even with the best of makeup removers. As well as Sorbolene, you can also use a water-based moisturiser under the eye to prevent staining.

Clumpy black mascara is hot with this look.

A high-shine luminescent foundation complements this look.

Use a translucent powder under the eye, below the black.

sexy eyes for redheads

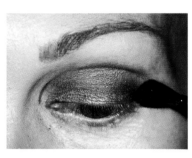

1 Prep the eyes. Using a medium brush, apply a purple wash over the whole eyelid, stopping just under the brow bone.

TIP

Make sure your brushes are very soft, and use a gentle motion. Harsh movements will create heavy lines, and make it harder to blend.

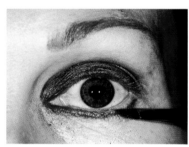

2 Using a wet angled brush, apply a copper pigment to the inner corners of the eye, top and bottom. Using the same brush (no need to clean it), apply an intense mahogany-red shadow under the bottom eyelashes, and in the inner corner of the eye, top and bottom.

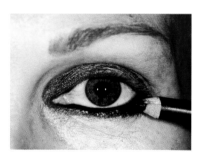

3 Line the eye rim heavily with a black non-waterproof eye pencil. This automatically changes the shape of the eye.

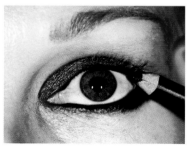

4 Line the upper rim of the eyelid heavily with the same non-waterproof black pencil.

5 Using a black shadow, heavily smudge the outer corner of the lid. Fill a clean medium brush with translucent powder, and use it to blend the black eye shadow and soften hard edges in an upward motion. This technique helps to extend the black into the outer corner of the eye.

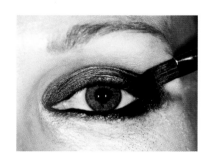

6 Clean up underneath the eye. The gentlest way to do this is to apply Sorbolene cream under the eye then use a wipe to remove any fallout.

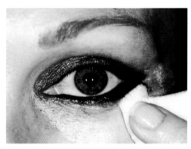

TIPS

Heavy black pigments are hard to find. A lot of them end up looking grey. If you have trouble finding one, use a cream black eyeliner or pencil.

A great idea before you start your lips is to load them up with lanolin or lip balm so they are moist for when you are ready to apply lipstick.

7 Curl lashes, and apply black mascara to the top and bottom lashes heavily (don't apply mascara if you are using false lashes—see the next step).

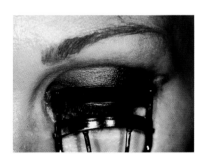

If you use too many products (eye cream, sunscreen etc.) around the eyes, the eye shadow will get cakey and heavy.

8 If you are using false lashes, apply a full set. Make sure they fit the eye correctly, and cut if necessary (for more information on applying lashes, refer to pages 32–40). Apply mascara. Notice the outer corner of the eye is not yet blended (blend after you apply your foundation).

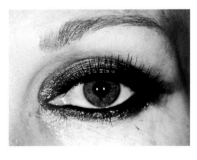

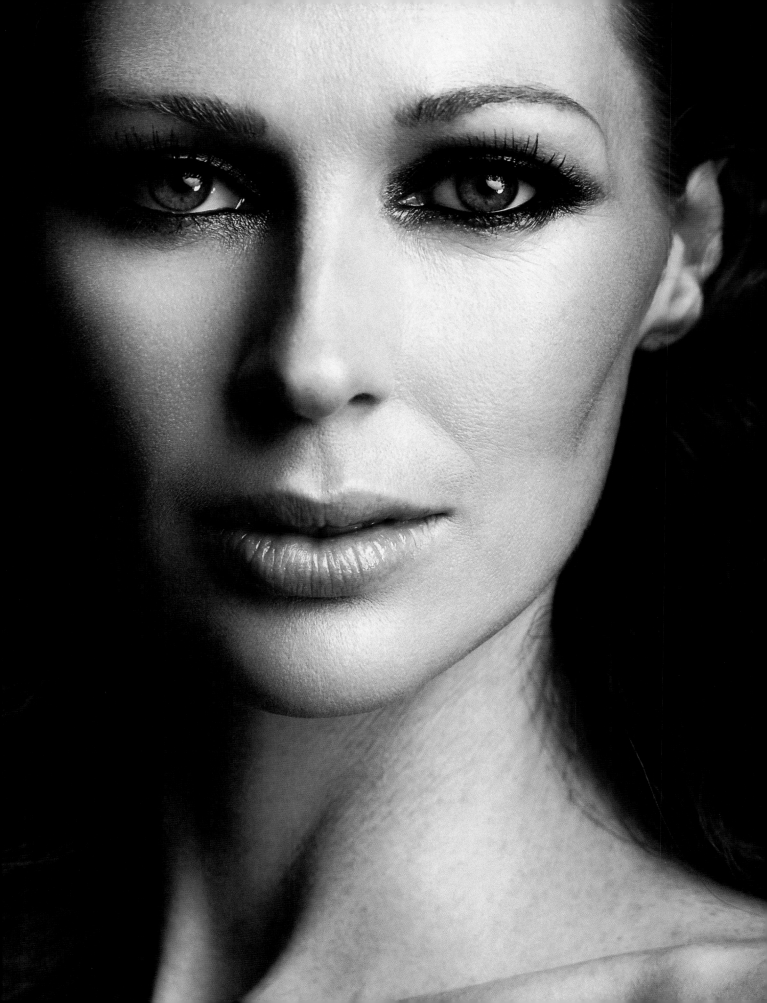

techno eyes

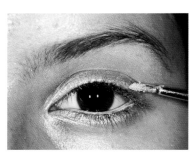

1 Prep the eyes and powder well. Using a fine brush, apply a soft metallic pale-gold shimmer powder over the entire eye, keeping it close to the lash line. Then apply a non-waterproof white pencil to the inner rim of the eye.

TIP

Gold leaf can be tricky as it sticks like glue. Only use a brush to pick it up from the packaging, otherwise it will stick to your fingers.

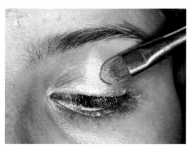

2 Using a medium brush, apply the same colour in the centre of the eyeball (as shown). This adds a beautiful highlight that will be visible when you blink.

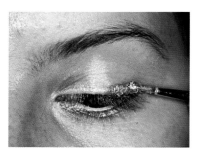

3 Using a wet fine brush, then apply a gold leaf (available from selected makeup stores and art shops) to the inner corner of the eye, and over the outer corner of the upper lid.

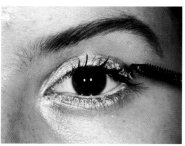

4 Curl lashes and apply a heavy amount of mascara to the top lashes only. Do not comb out your lashes, keep them clumpy.

70

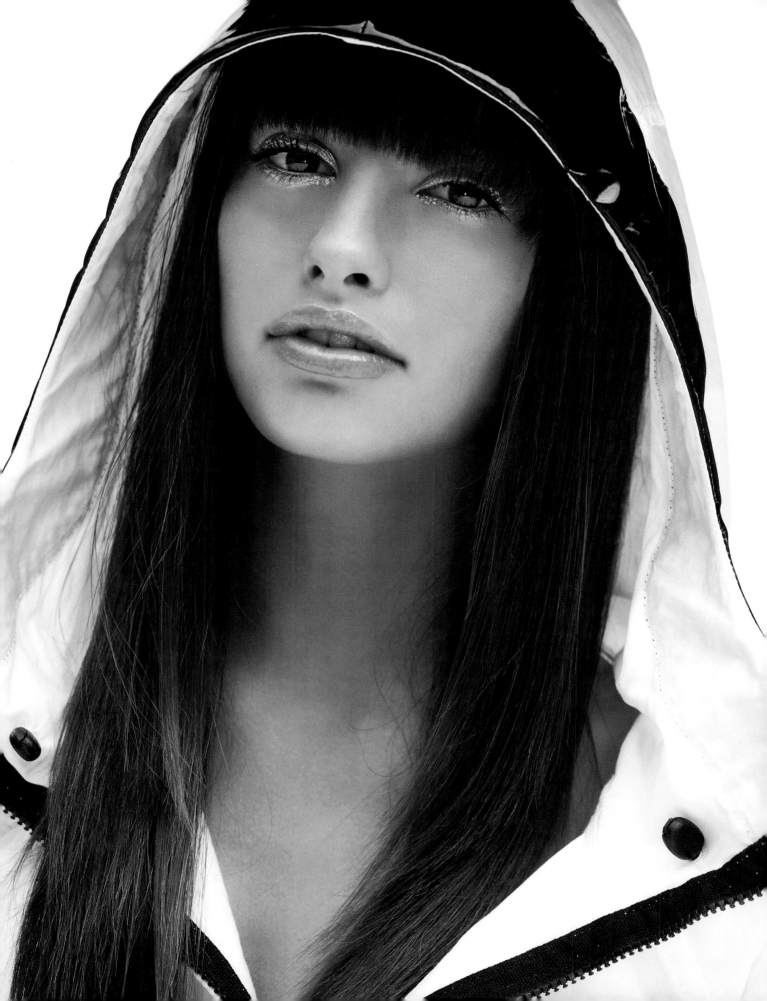

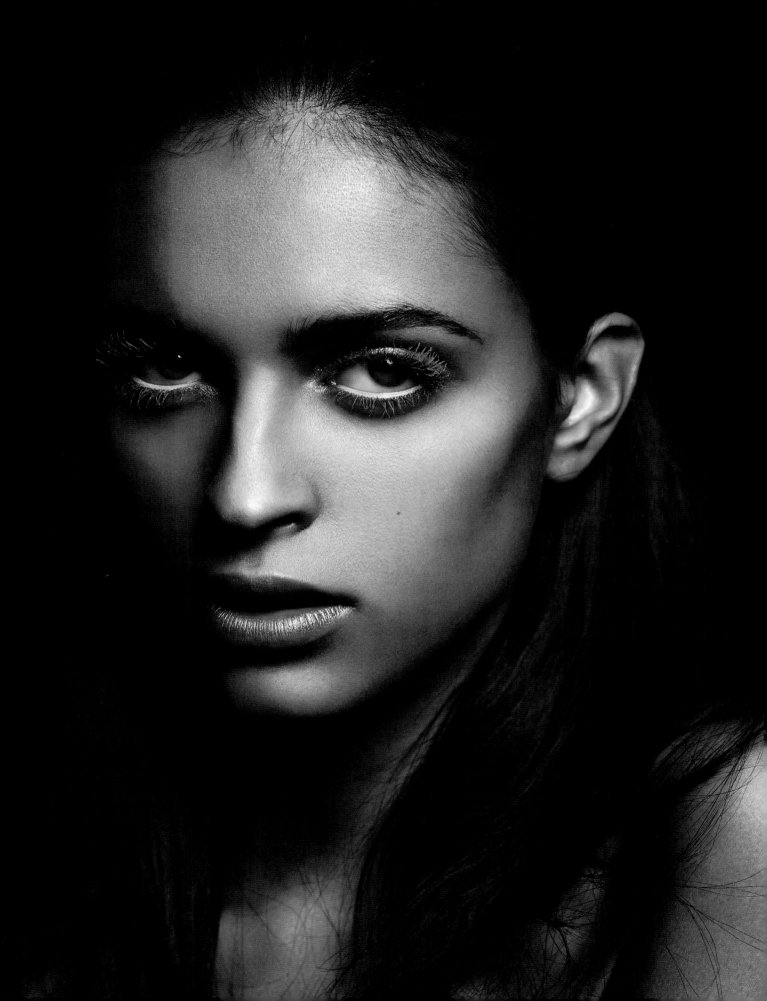

turquoise evening eyes

1 Using a medium brush, apply a soft mint-green wash to the whole eyelid, to just underneath the brow bone. Remember, this will blend easily if your eyelids are prepped and powdered.

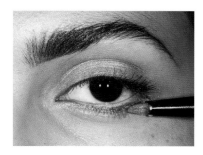

2 Using a thin brush, apply the same colour under the length of the bottom lash line. The colour must stay very close to the lash line, because if you let metallic colours drop too low it will look like you haven't slept in weeks, make fine lines look worse and have a scaling effect.

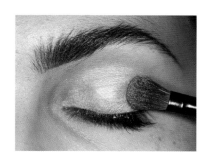

TIP

With this look, tone down blush so that it's virtually undetectable. This is a great look for low-light locations, awesome on dark-coloured eyes and all blue-toned eyes.

3 Apply a white pencil heavily to the inner rim of the eye. This makes your eyes look whiter, wider and more alive. Using a thin brush, apply a strong electric-blue pigment along the top and bottom outer lash line. Don't worry about fallout—fix it later.

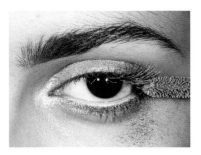

4 Curl lashes, and apply an intense amount of turquoise mascara. Using a fine angled brush, highlight the inner corners with soft iridescent silver.

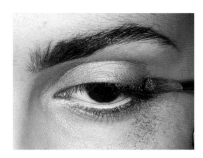

electric blue eyes

TIPS

The smaller the area you're working on, the smaller the brush should be.

Pale blue eye shadow can be very scary. If used incorrectly, it can look cheap and nasty. I believe most frosty eye shadow needs depth and intensity to look beautiful, so use a little black or a darker version of the colour you choose. With Michelle's eyebrows, I filled them in lightly to give more definition.

For step 3, you can also use black eye shadow along the lash line to make the colour more intense.

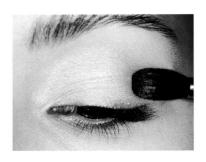

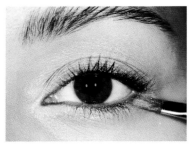

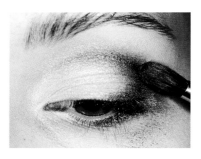

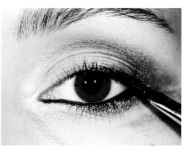

1 Prep the eyes and apply a soft wash of translucent powder. Using a medium brush, apply a soft, iridescent blue eye shadow to the whole eyelid and blend up to the brow bone.

2 Using a small brush, apply the same colour all the way along the bottom of the eye. Make sure you use very light pressure; this will guarantee a smooth, even result. It helps to look up while doing this because it stretches the skin and stops unwanted lines from appearing.

3 Using a medium brush, apply a midnight-blue shadow to create depth. Blend lightly under the brow bone and apply one-third of the way along the lash line. This should be the darkest point of the eye. Make sure to avoid gaps of bare skin and don't put too much pressure on the brush, as you will create fine lines.

4 Apply a midnight-blue eye pencil, or cream eyeliner, heavily to the inner rim of the eye, and to the outer corner of the lid. This lifts the eye and makes it look younger and more cat-like. It also frames the eye, giving it more definition. Finish by applying mascara.

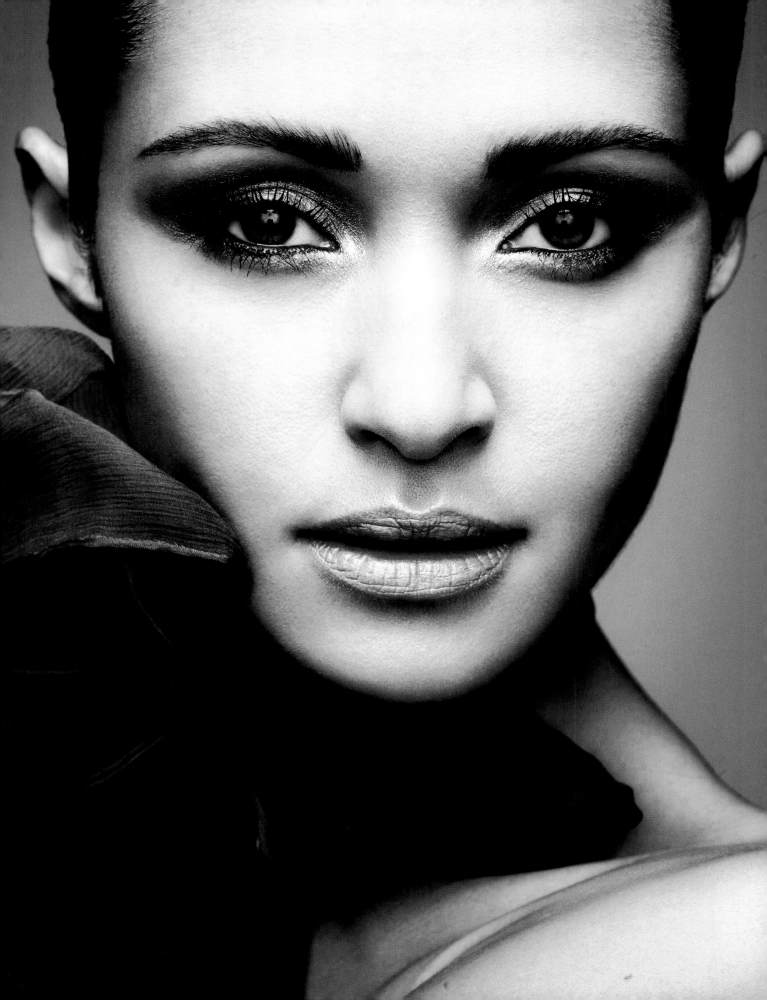

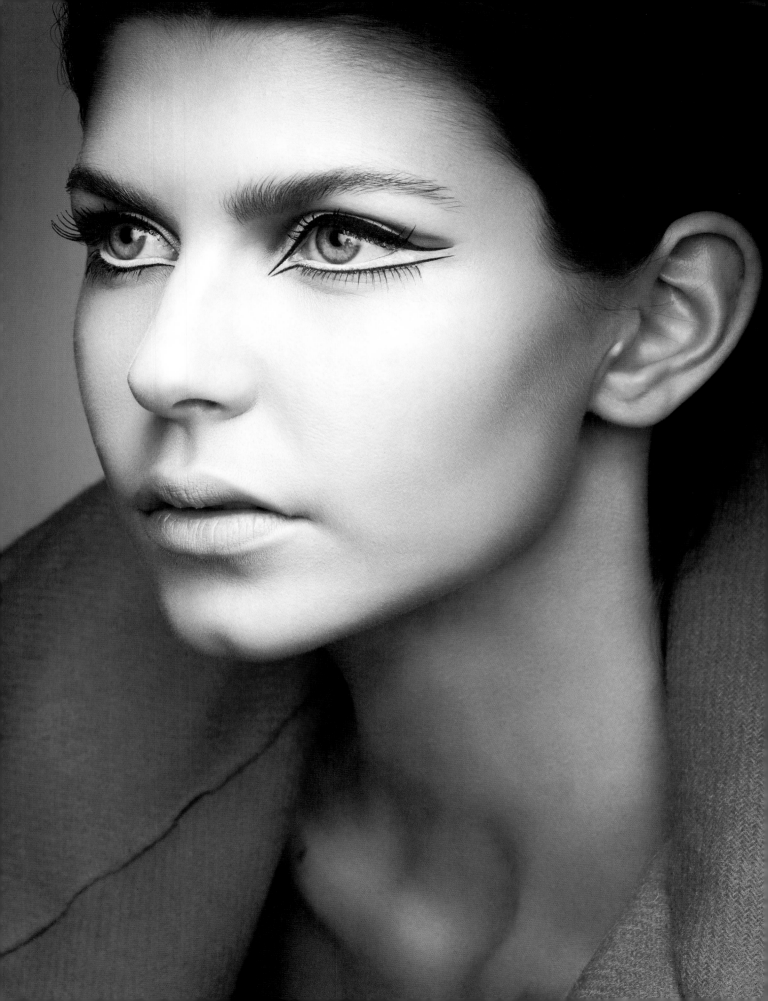

retro eyes

1 Lightly foundation the eyelid, but do not powder yet. Using a medium brush, apply white water-based liquid eye paint to the lid. Keep looking down while waiting for the paint to dry, otherwise it will crease. To set this, use a white eye shadow over the dried paint.

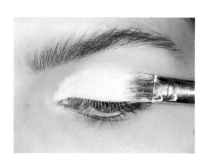

TIPS

The reason I am using a paint before the eye shadow is because eye shadows on their own don't give a strong enough intensity. You need to have the paint base to make the white stand out more. This is one of the most difficult looks to achieve. It will take at least half an hour to do.

Use a non-waterproof pencil on the inner rim of the eye because it is a wet area. A waterproof pencil will scratch the skin and will not work.

2 Heavily apply a white eye pencil to the inner rim of the eye. This needs to be non-waterproof to ensure an intense colour. Extend the white line straight out past the outer corner of the eye and create a triangle to the inner corner (as shown).

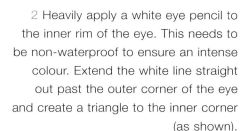

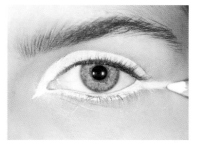

3 Using a stiff angled brush, apply black eye shadow above the eyelid (don't use a fine eyeliner brush). Extend the line out from the edge of the lid. Eyeliner looks its best when the line thickens towards the outer socket.

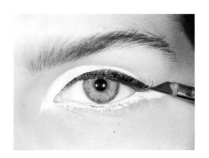

4 Using black eye shadow and a slightly wet angled brush, draw a line underneath the eye as shown, making sure you are looking directly ahead to ensure a straight line.

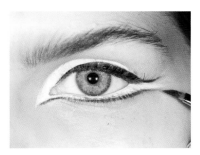

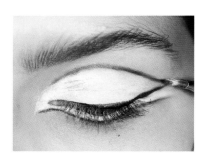

5 Extend the line above the top lash line up and out. Draw another thin line following the crease in the eyelid, moving from the inner to the outer, connecting to the line above the lid in the shape of a V.

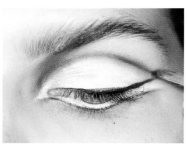

6 Using a thin brush, slightly blend the line into the crease in your lid.

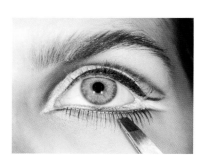

7 I am using clear eyelash glue on the bottom false lashes before applying mascara, which I rarely do. Apply a full set of lashes along the line you have created under the eye.

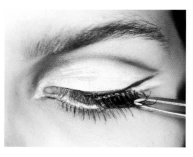

8 Apply a full set of false lashes to the top lash line, gluing it to the line you have already created with the eyeliner. Finish by applying mascara.

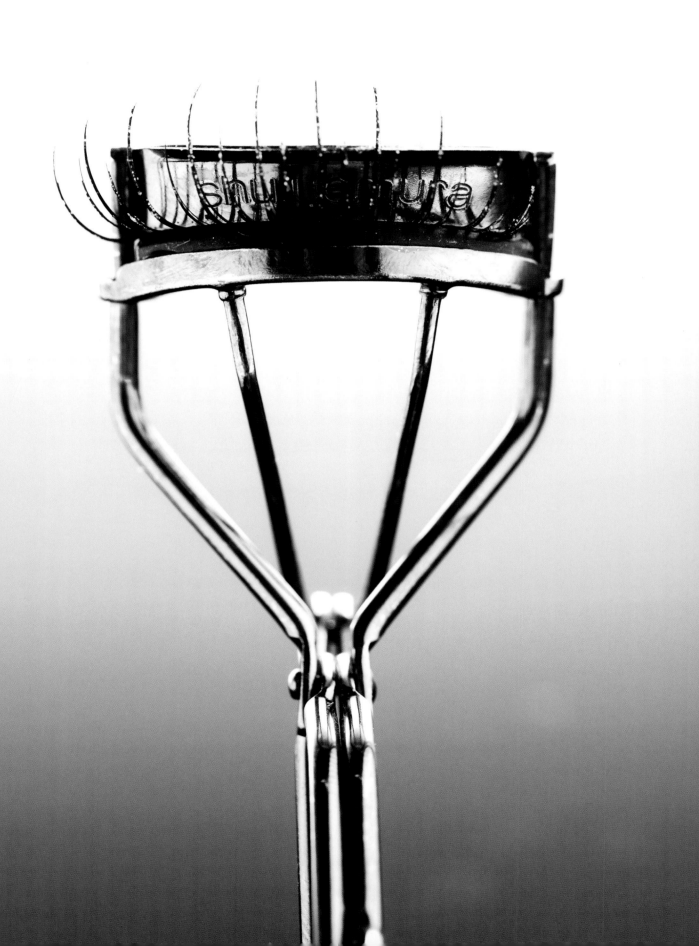

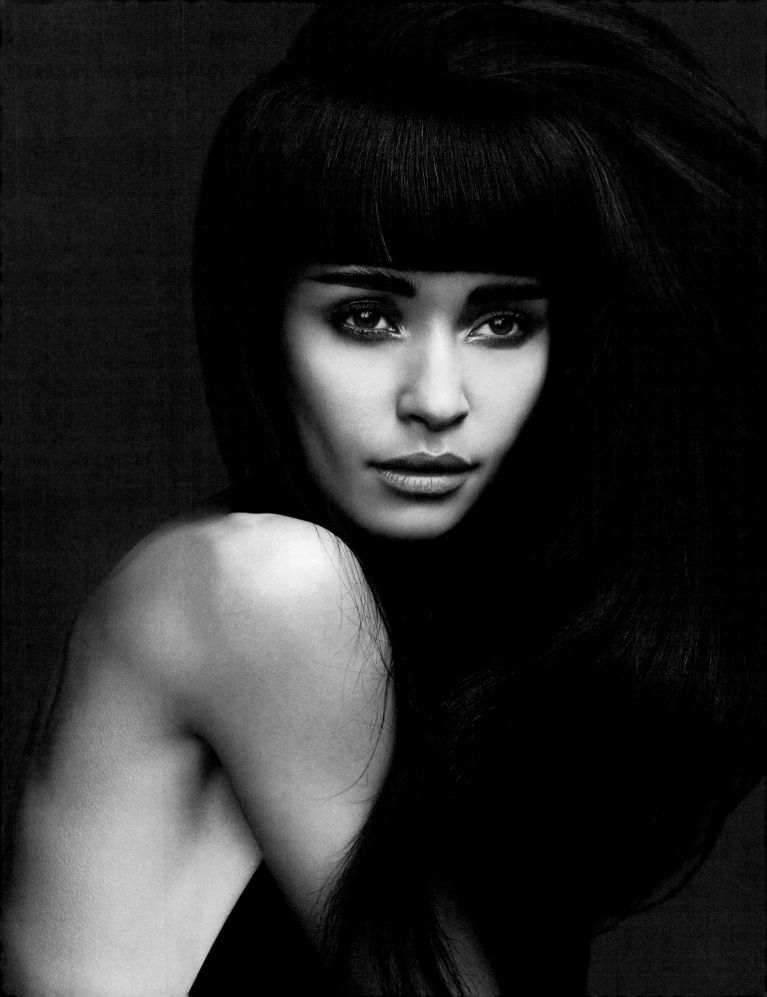

harajuku eyes

1 Create a stencil with sticky tape (use soft, magic tape which is easy to remove) directly under the eyebrow, to create a straight line (as shown).

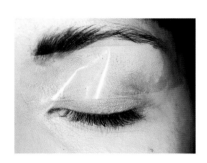

2 Use a deep-red eye shadow to draw in the area above the stencil line, to recreate the eyebrow. Then using a thin brush, apply a strong orange pigment along the brow line. Do not blend with the eye shadow. Then remove the tape.

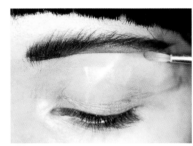

3 Using a large brush (for easy blending), apply a cream khaki-coloured eye shadow all over lid. Do not extend it to the brow bone.

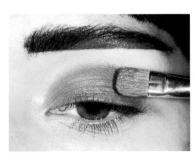

4 Apply gold eyeliner to the inner rim of the eye, and finish up with a coat of mascara. You can use mascara on the top and bottom lashes to keep a more rounded shape.

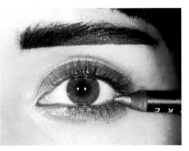

TIPS

To contrast with the shiny eyelids, I have used a sheer powder on the face—you don't want shiny skin with shiny eyes.

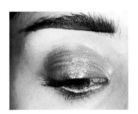

I've included this shot especially to show the problems created with grease and cream shadows. This shot was taken 10 minutes after makeup was applied; see how quickly the eye shadow has creased? Magazines are filled with wet, sexy-looking eyes, but these have a lasting ability of only 10 minutes. So only use if you are ready to constantly smooth it out.

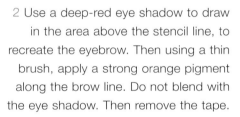

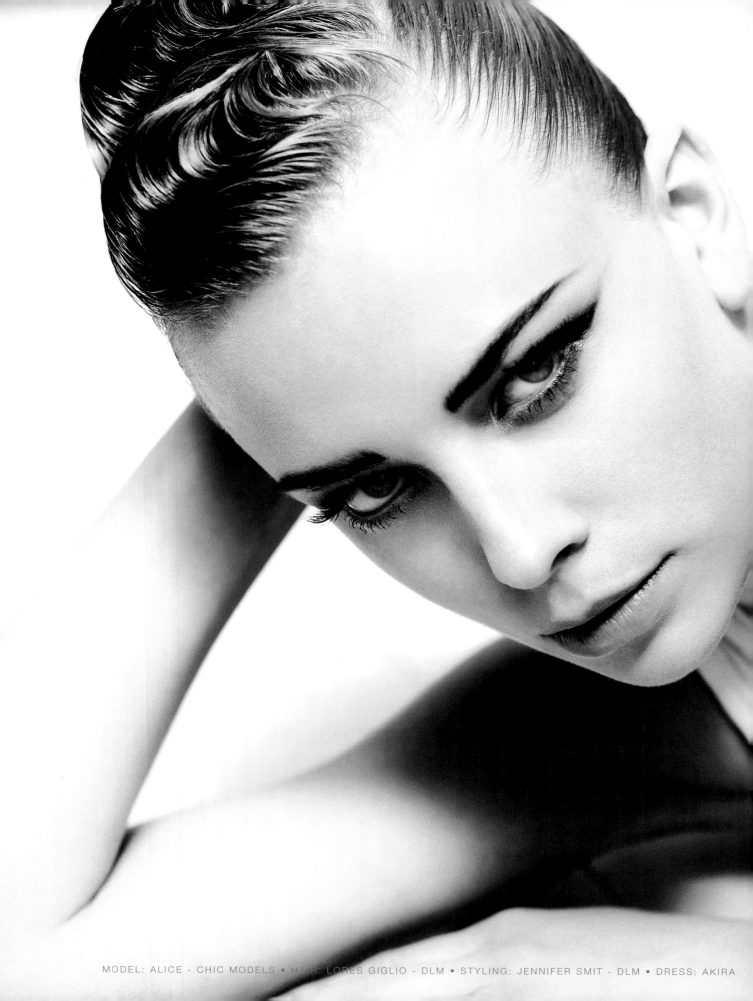

exotic eyes

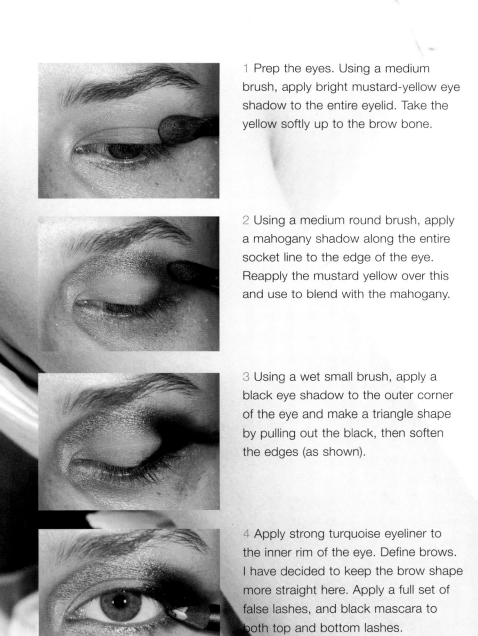

1 Prep the eyes. Using a medium brush, apply bright mustard-yellow eye shadow to the entire eyelid. Take the yellow softly up to the brow bone.

2 Using a medium round brush, apply a mahogany shadow along the entire socket line to the edge of the eye. Reapply the mustard yellow over this and use to blend with the mahogany.

3 Using a wet small brush, apply a black eye shadow to the outer corner of the eye and make a triangle shape by pulling out the black, then soften the edges (as shown).

4 Apply strong turquoise eyeliner to the inner rim of the eye. Define brows. I have decided to keep the brow shape more straight here. Apply a full set of false lashes, and black mascara to both top and bottom lashes.

TIP
Because this is such a strong and unique look, make sure you match it with prominent brows.

egyptian eyes

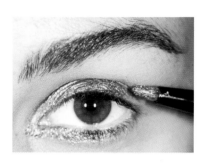

1 Using a wet small brush, apply a mahogany, deep chocolate-brown eye shadow underneath the eye and over the top lid, keeping the intensity in the inner corner.

TIP

Mahogany is the only colour in the colour wheel that is both cool and warm. It is suitable for any time of day and with any look. Gemma's brows are beautifully arched, however, to give a sexier, more polished look. Make the brows less rounded for a straighter look.

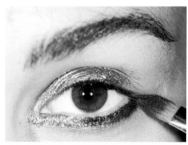

2 Using a small brush, apply the same shadow under the rim of the eye, then pull it out slightly to the outer edge of the eye to create a smudged eyeliner.

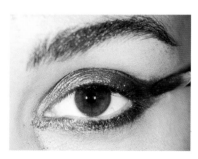

3 Turn your brush upside down, and apply the same shadow to the top lid. This will keep the intensity along the lash line (this will eliminate the mistake of leaving skin gaps). Apply more shadow to keep it heavier on the outer corner of the top lid.

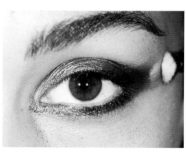

4 Apply a bit of loose translucent powder, making sure it matches your skin tone. In Gemma's case, I am using a yellow tone. Curl the lashes, and apply lots of mascara to top and bottom lashes. Clean up under the eye, and apply foundation.

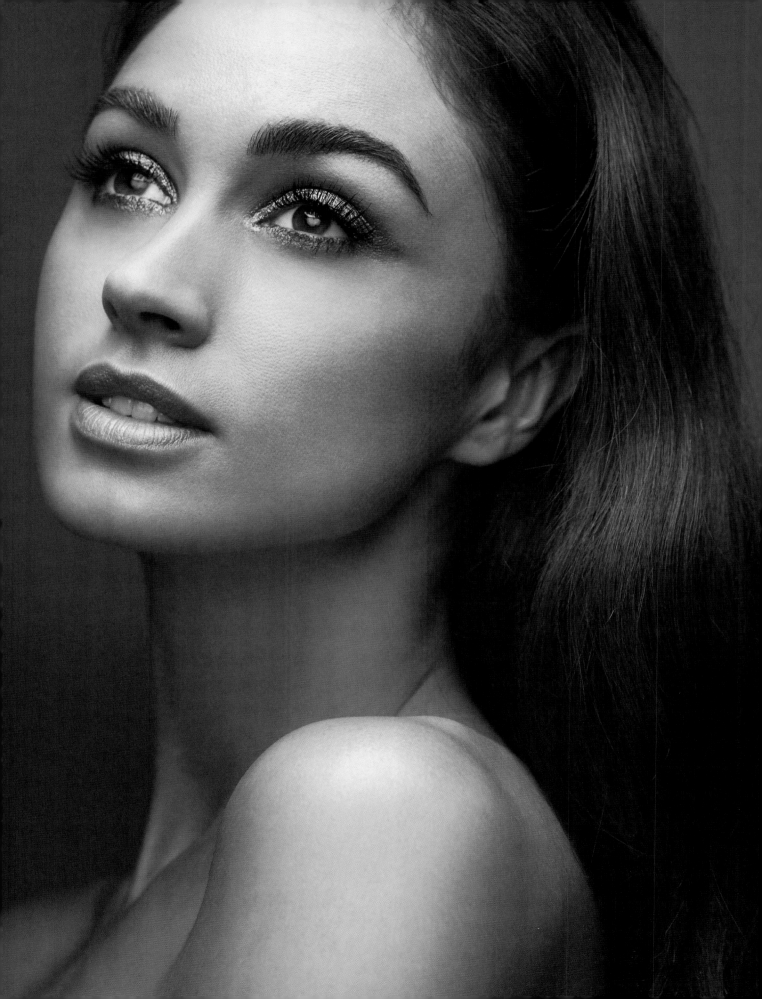

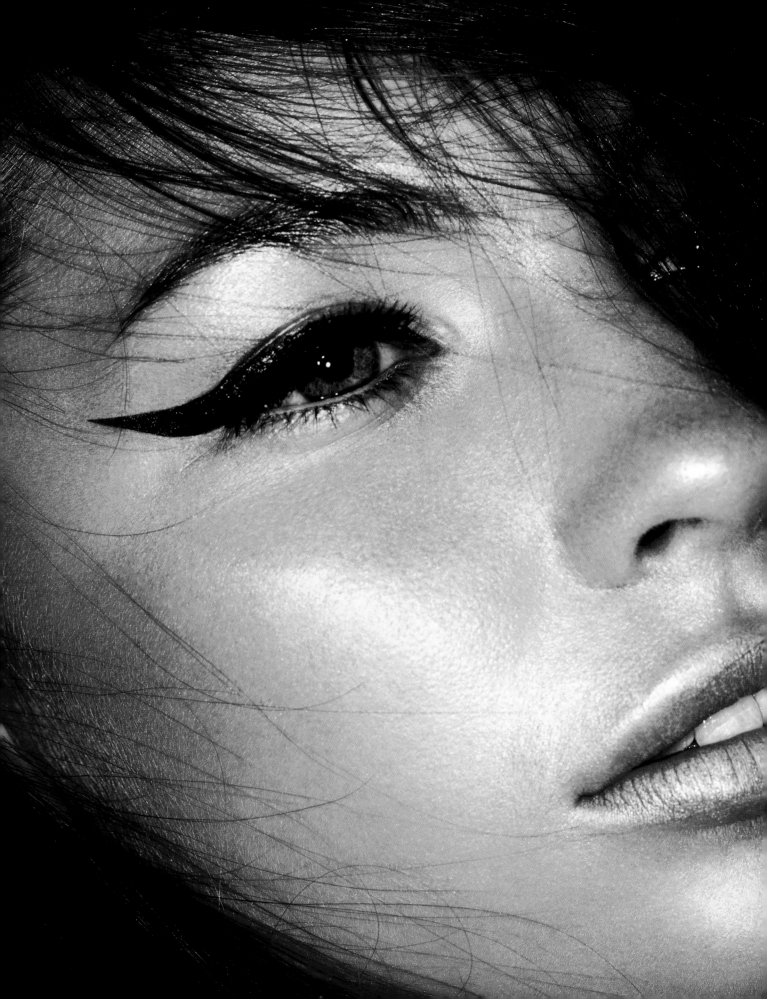

cat-like eyes

1 Imagine a line from the corner of your nose to the outer corner of your eye that continues to your temple. Your eyeliner needs to follow this angle. Apply sticky tape as a stencil on that angle. Using a small angled brush, apply black liquid liner along your lash line, flicking up onto the tape.

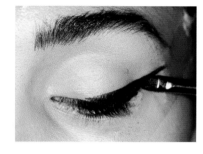

2 Wait for the liner to dry, then carefully peel off the tape. Apply a bright blue pigment on the inner corner of the eye, to meet the liquid liner.

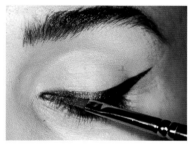

TIPS

The sticky tape will ensure your line is straight.

If you wish, you can use black eye shadow instead of the liquid liner.

3 Curl lashes and apply lots of mascara to the top lashes only; make sure the mascara is applied all the way to the bed of the lashes.

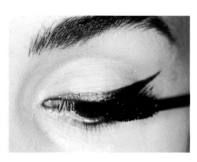

4 Apply false lashes to the top eyelid. Finish the look by applying foundation and a light metallic lipstick.

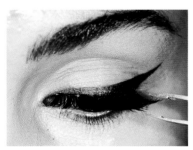

aqua eyes

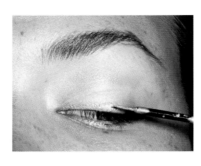

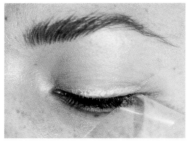

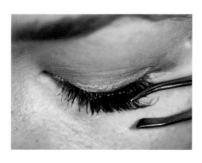

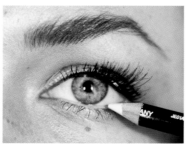

TIPS

This is one of the few dramatic eye looks where you can do the foundation first. Then use an alcohol-free baby wipe to remove oil from the eyelid. This will stop the eyeliner from bleeding.

Most liquid eyeliners tend to crack, so choose gel or cream liners instead. These will give you time to move and blend before they dry.

1 Prep your eyes and lightly powder. I am breaking the eyeliner into two sections. Using an eyeliner brush, apply an aqua-green eyeliner from the inside of the eyelid, stopping in the centre. This will stretch the skin and minimise wrinkles and creasing in the lid.

2 Apply sticky tape as a stencil on an imaginary angle, from the corner of your nose to the outer corner of your eye. Then finish applying the eyeliner from the centre to the upper outer edge as shown. The sticky tape will ensure you get a perfect line.

3 Curl lashes and apply lots of black mascara to the top and bottom lashes. Make sure the mascara is jet-black. Then apply a full lash that has been cut in half to the top lashes only (see the False Eyelashes chapter, page 30).

4 Apply non-waterproof white eyeliner to the inner rim of the eye. This will open up the eye and make it look more alive.

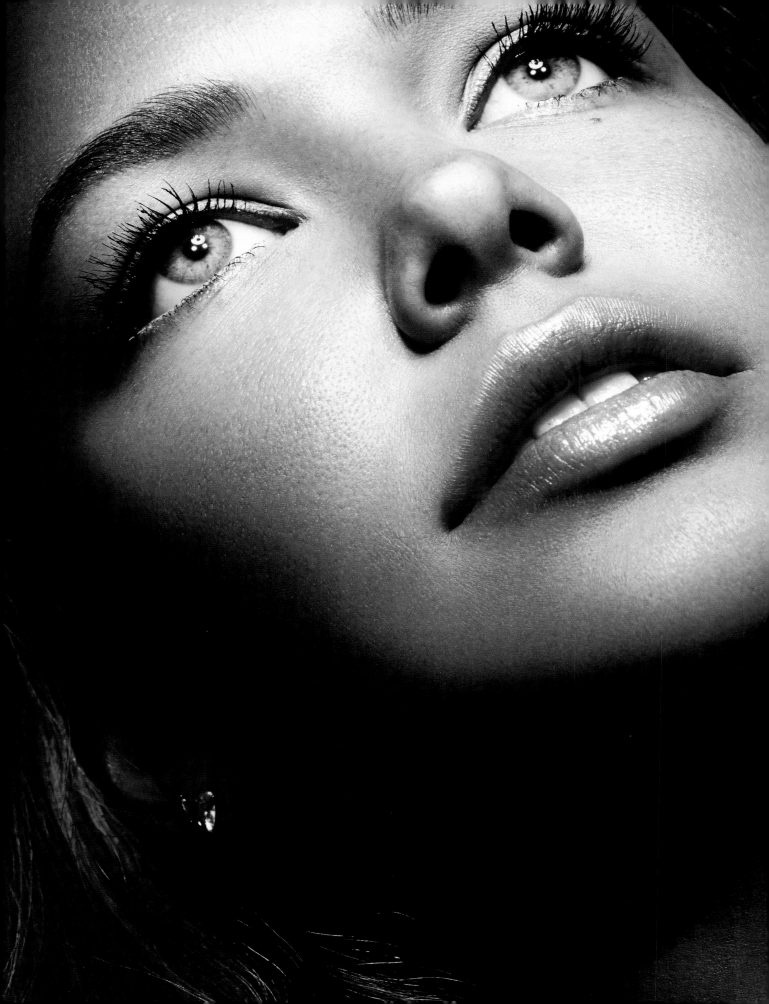

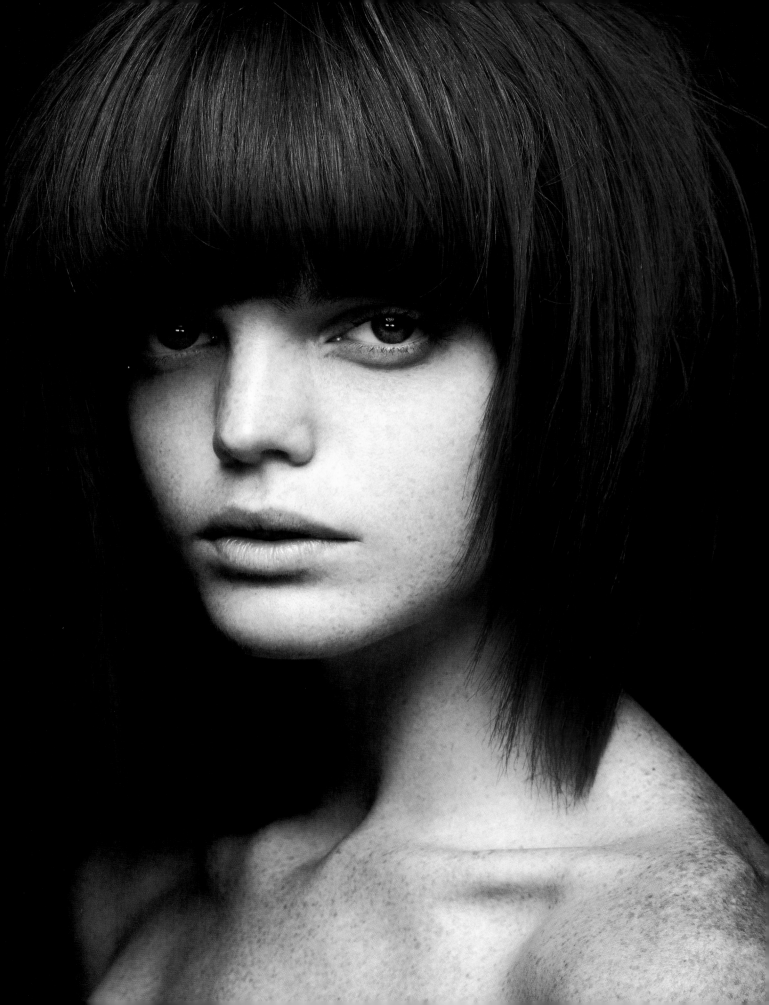

antique gold eyes

1 Clean up the brows. Prep the eye with foundation, but no powder. (You don't powder because you are applying the pigment with a wet brush, and powder will only make the pigment coagulate). Using a medium brush, apply an antique gold shadow to the entire lid.

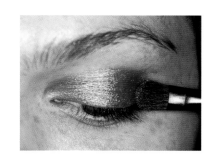

2 Continue the same gold pigment to the inner corner of the eye. Then apply an intense gold eyeliner to the inner rim and along the top eyelash line.

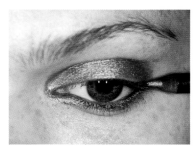

TIP

This is not the easiest of looks to achieve, so give yourself plenty of time to practise before you try it for an evening out. These eyes must be finished off with beautifully defined brows, otherwise the look doesn't seem finished.

3 Using a wet thin brush, apply a thin layer of cream blue-black pigment by drawing a diagonal line from the inner corner of the eye to the brow. The line should cut through the brow bone.

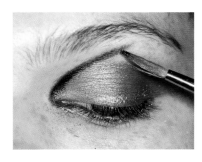

4 Using an angled brush, apply the blue-black pigment to the crease of the eye, following your natural socket line, beginning at the top and working downwards in a straight line. The line should end in line with the end of your brow. A steady hand is essential!

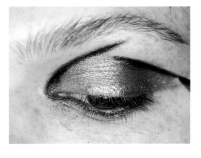

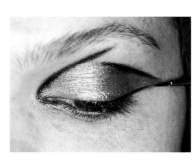

5 Extend the antique gold eye shadow into a triangular shape, then apply a very fine deep-blue eyeliner along the outer top lash line, and extend it out slightly.

LASHES USED

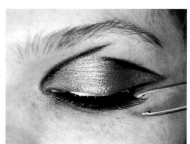

6 Curl lashes and apply a full set of false lashes. Notice I have applied a light-feathery lash as opposed to a heavy lash.

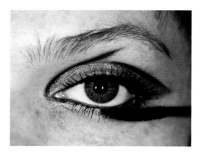

7 Apply black mascara to both the real and fake lashes to give a thicker effect. Make it slightly clumpy if you wish. This look is great for light-coloured lashes. Apply a gel blue-black eyeliner along the top lash line.

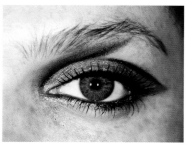

8 To soften the black line that extends from the inner corner to the brow bone, use a soft black eye shadow and lightly blend over it.

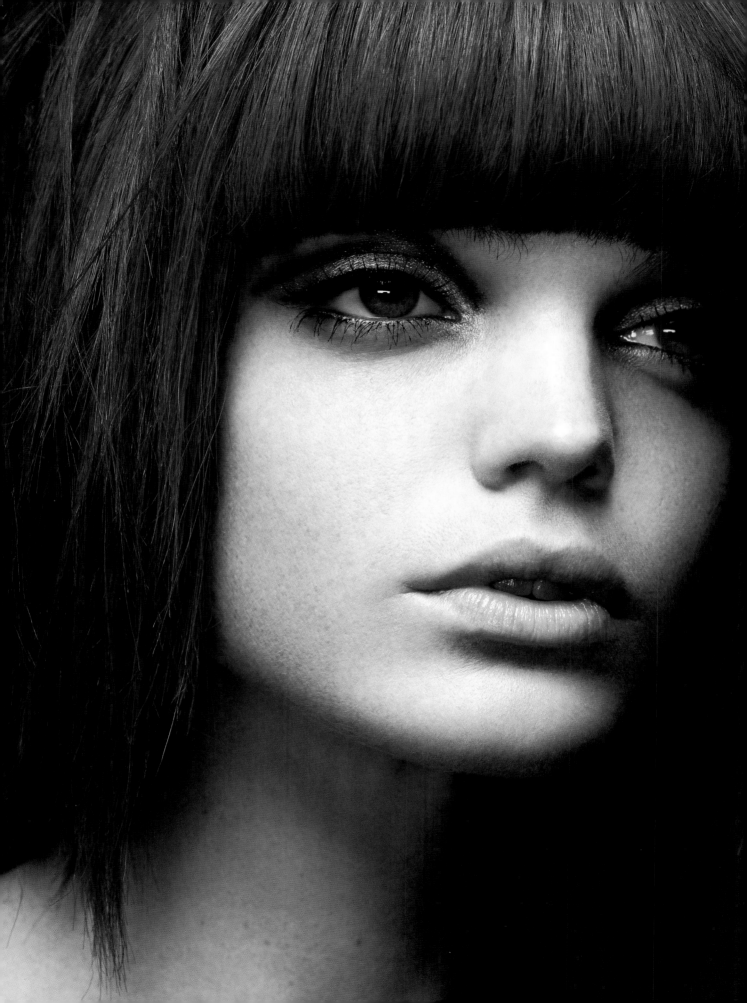

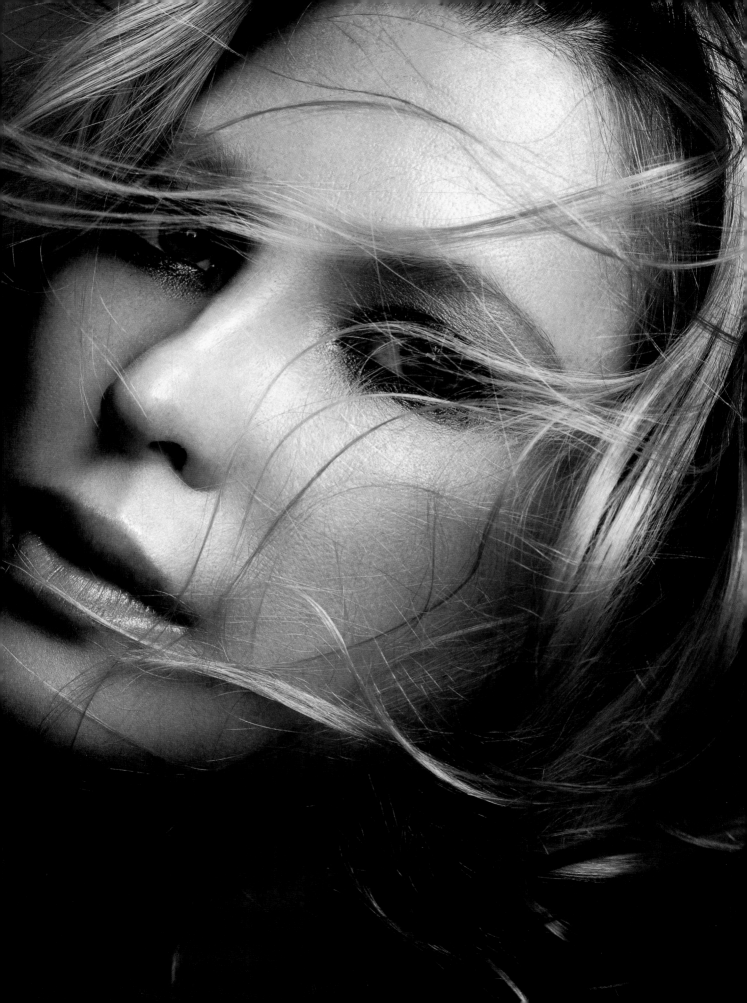

sensual eyes

1 Prep your eye then, using a medium brush, apply a golden copper pigment under the eye. Note that it's a few millimetres wide so that when you apply the darker shade it has something to blend out to.

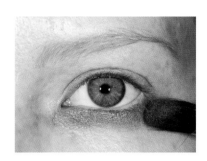

2 Apply the same pigment around the entire eye, carrying it up to the brow. Then apply a chocolate-brown metallic pencil to the inner rim of the eye (a matt brown pencil is also a great option).

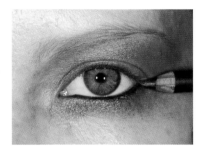

3 Using a thin brush, apply a dark mahogany brown to the upper lid, concentrating along the lash line. Note the shape is straight across the lid, not rounded. Apply this under the eye as well, intensifying it near the outer edge.

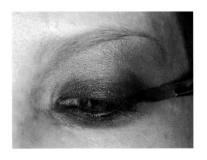

4 Finish by applying a black pigment around the eye, close to the lash line. Then add mascara to the top and bottom lashes.

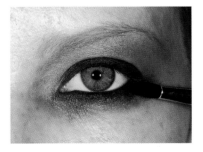

burnt copper eyes

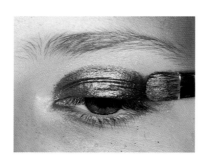

1 Using a wet medium brush, apply copper pigment on the eyelid only. (Wetting the brush intensifies the colour and stops fallout.)

TIP

I have used electric-blue eye shadow because it is the opposite of orange. I wanted to add a contrasting colour to make it stand out as orange is overpowering, and any other colour wouldn't be noticed.

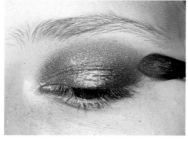

2 Apply a light translucent orange powder above the copper to help you blend. Use a pointed, flexible, soft brush for easier blending. You can also load up your brush with translucent powder to help the process.

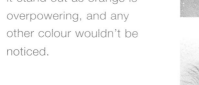

LASHES USED

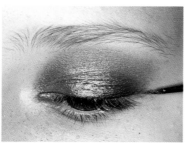

3 Using a wet thin brush, apply an electric-blue eye shadow very finely along the top lash line. Leave no gaps between the lash line and the blue liner.

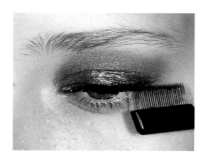

4 Curl lashes and apply black mascara. A great technique to separate the lashes without clumps is to use a lash comb as shown. Alternatively, use an old mascara wand from a previous mascara (washed, of course!).

96

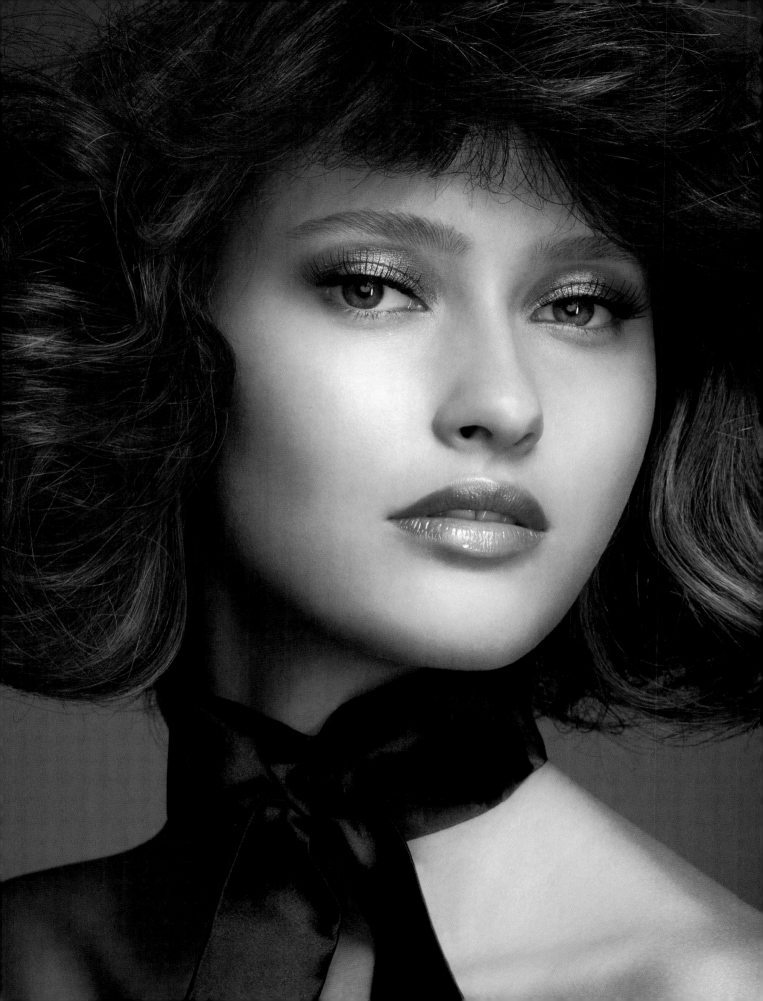

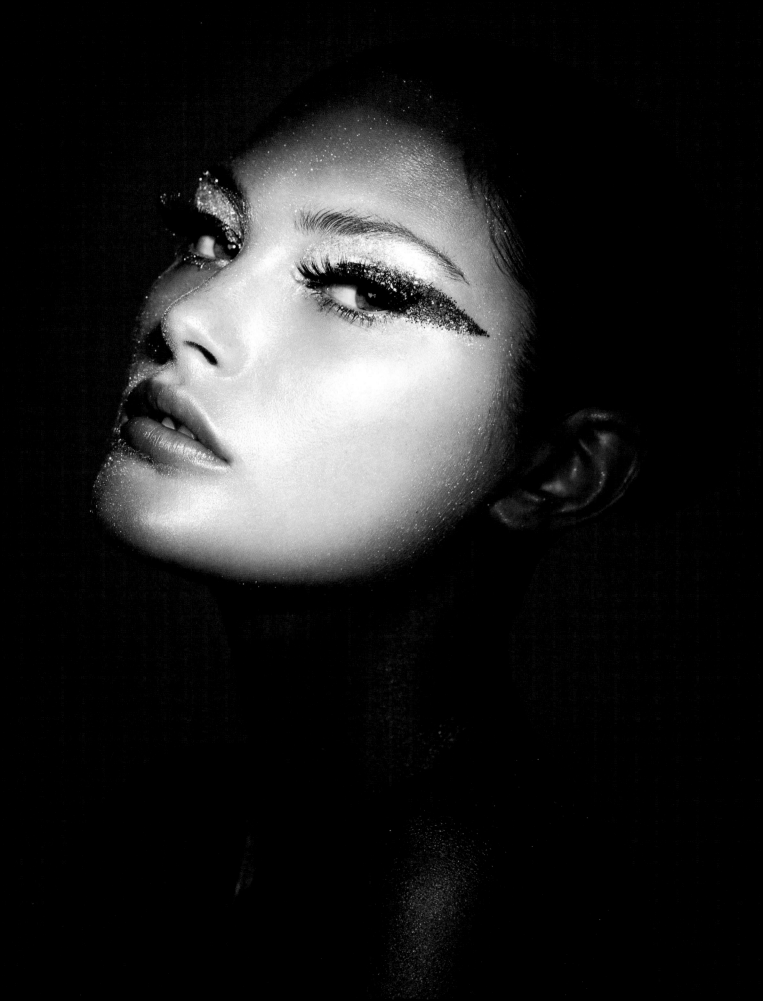

cleopatra eyes

1 Apply powder to all the places around the eye where the glitter is *not* meant to go: the brow bone, inner eye rim, beneath the eye and so on.

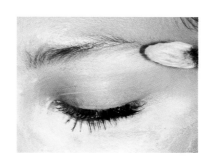

2 Paint eyelash glue on the eyelid. Only use a brush that you don't mind waving goodbye to. Wait until the glue is sticky and tacky before you apply the glitter, and only do one eye at a time, as getting glue in the eye can be very dangerous.

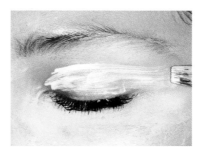

TIPS

Remember, only put eyelash glue where you want the glitter eye shadow to go.

I've finished off the look by dusting Catherine's skin with silver shimmer powder.

LASHES USED

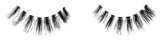

3 Using a medium brush, apply the charcoal or gunmetal-grey glitter evenly over the glue. Use a small hairdryer to blow off unwanted glitter.

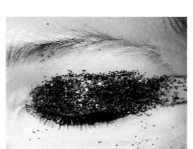

4 Use masking tape to gently remove unwanted glitter remnants. Then use a cotton pad with Sorbolene cream to clean up under the eye. Gently wipe off any excess powder, and finish with foundation and mascara.

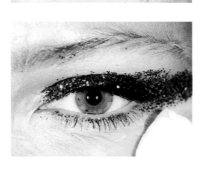

diva eyes

TIP
This look requires well-defined brows. You should clean up your brows before you prep your eyes.

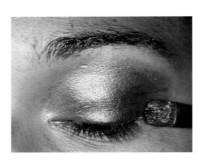

1 Prep the eye but don't powder. Wet your brush and apply a rose-gold pigment over the whole lid. Then apply a strong copper pigment over the lid but not as high as the first colour. This will blend the two colours beautifully. Don't look up for 1 minute to avoid creasing.

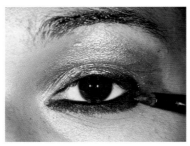

2 Apply a creamy black eyeliner to the inner lash rim and along one-third of the top lash line. Make sure this is smudged into the lash line, so there are no skin-coloured gaps along the lower lash line. It may look heavy at this stage, but you need this depth to create the eye shape.

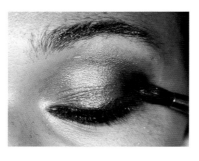

3 Using a wet brush, apply black pigment to the outer corner of the eye and smudge. This creates depth and drama, and is great for small or closely set eyes.

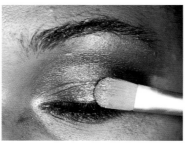

4 Apply an antique gold shadow heavily to the inner corner V of the eye, and smack bang in the middle of the eyelid. Also apply on the brow bone just under the eyebrow.

5 Define the brows. Curl the lashes and apply plenty of black mascara to the top and bottom lashes. Use a very strong false lash with eyelash glue.

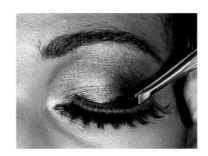

6 Apply lip balm to moisturise your lips and act as a base. Then apply pigment over the entire lips. Note that I'm using a metallic pigment as a lipstick. This is a good way to get strong lips, as most lipsticks will not give you this intensity.

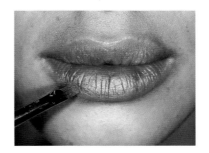

TIP
I am using black eyelash glue here to apply the false lashes. You can use white glue, but you may need a fair amount so it may take a while to dry.

7 Take the same antique gold used on the eye, and apply to the cupid's bow of the lips, and the middle of the bottom lip. I rarely recommend that women apply makeup using cotton buds, but they are perfect for applying the gold to the middle of the bottom lip.

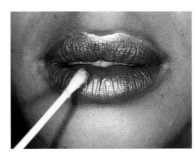

LASHES USED

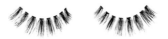

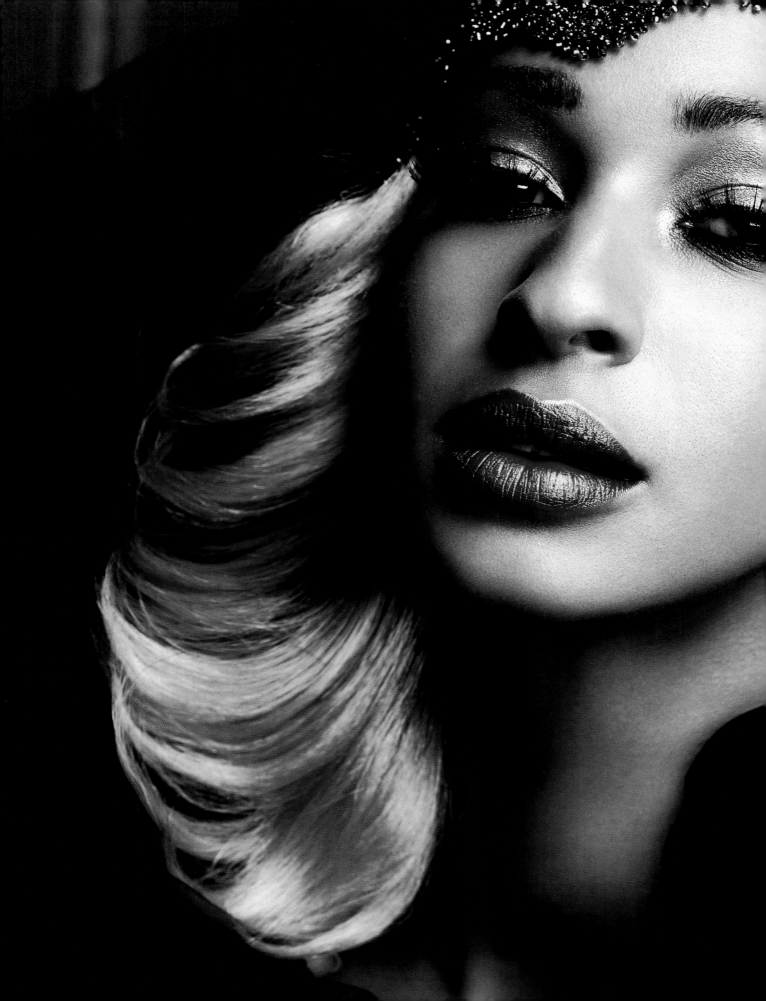

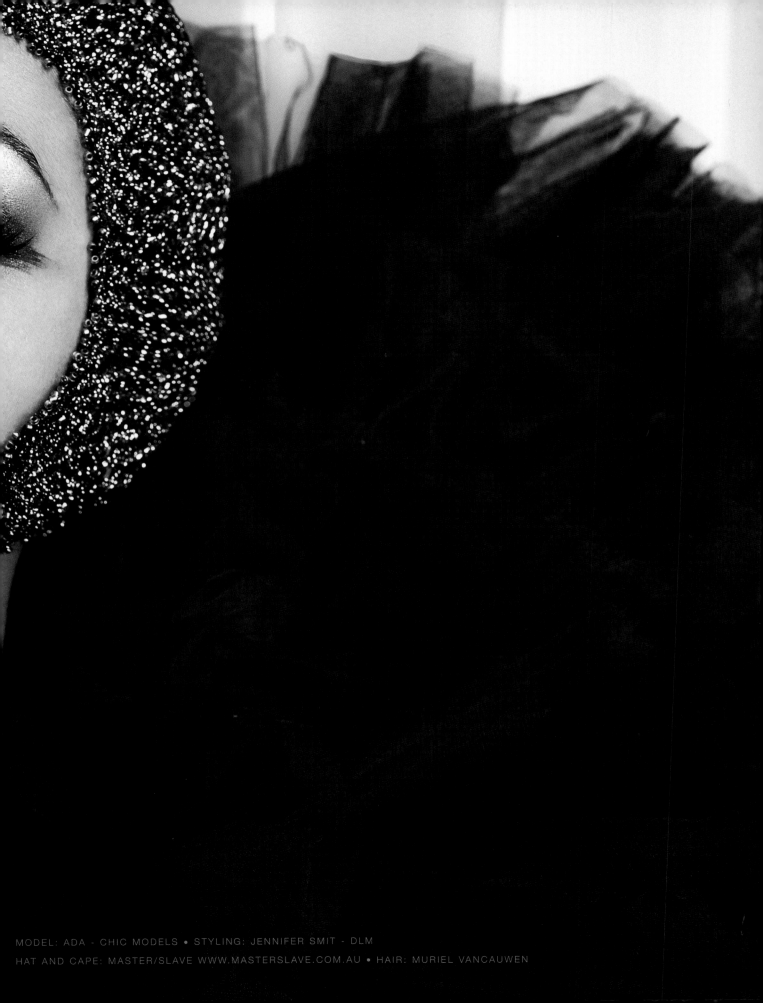

MODEL: ADA - CHIC MODELS • STYLING: JENNIFER SMIT - DLM
HAT AND CAPE: MASTER/SLAVE WWW.MASTERSLAVE.COM.AU • HAIR: MURIEL VANCAUWEN

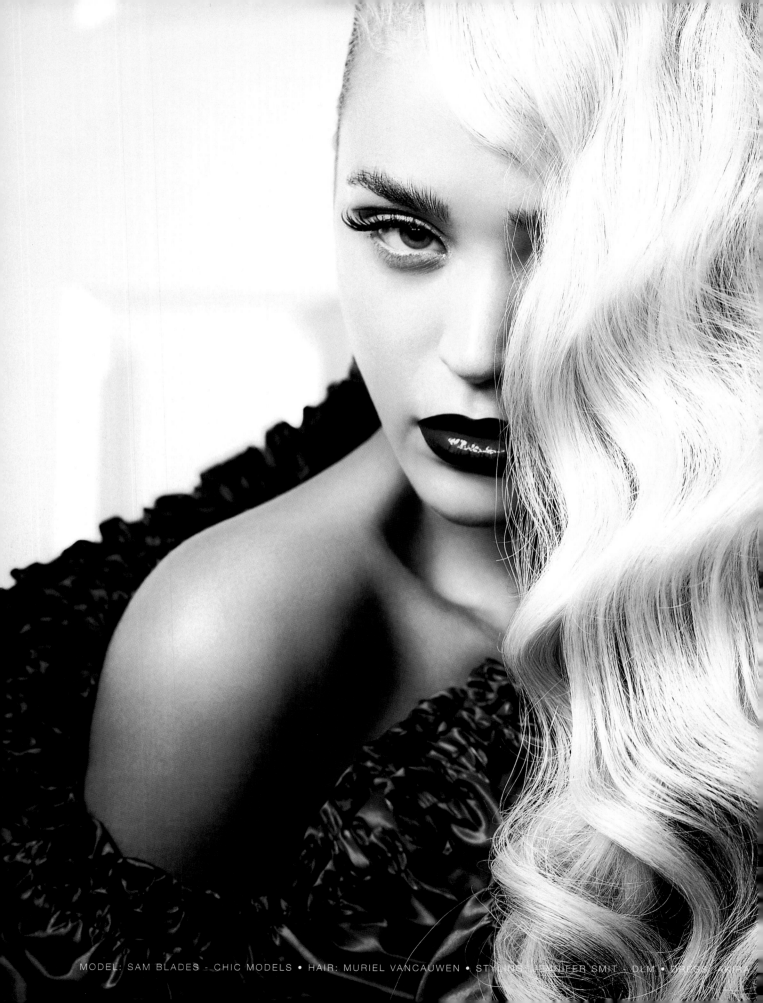

lilac eyes

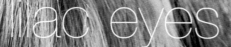

1 Using a medium brush, apply a soft wash of lavender to the eyelid, then add a little bit of white wash to the centre of the eyelid.

2 Starting from the inner eye socket, just under the brow bone, apply navy-black eye shadow in a fine line following the arch of the eyelid.

3 Clean up the fallout from the liner on the upper lid, by using a small brush with lavender eye shadow to blend.

4 Comb brows. Wet your brush and apply a white frost pigment. Make sure the colour is translucent, to allow the original lavender colour to show through. Also apply heavily to the inner corner of the eye. Curl lashes and apply plenty of black mascara to the top lashes only.

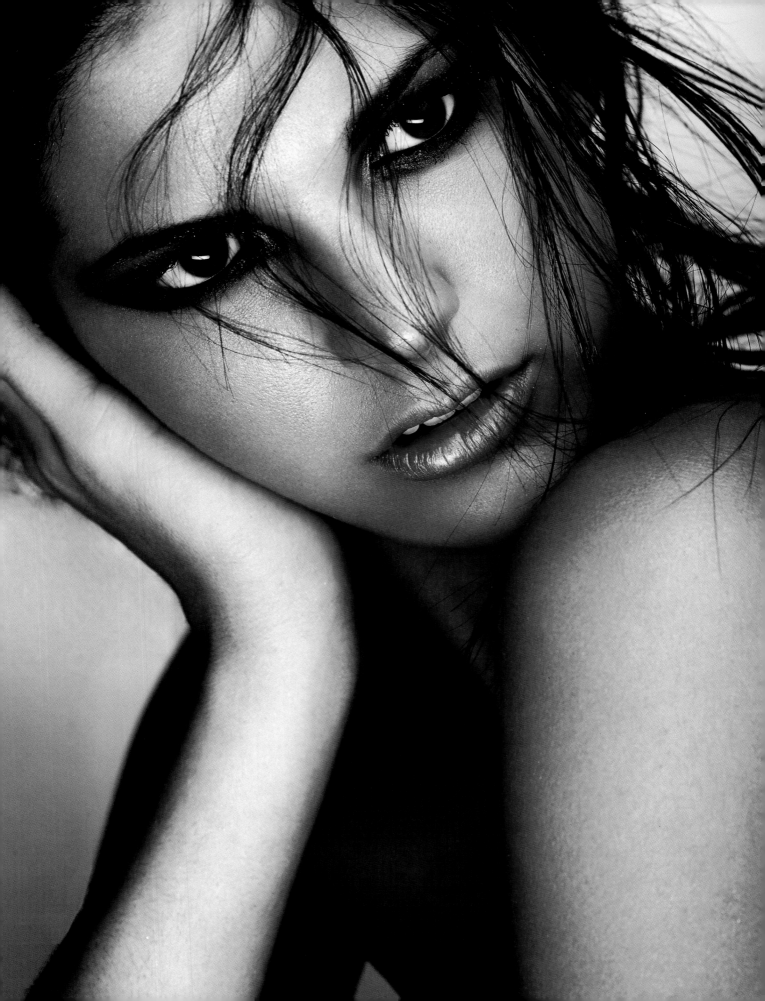

smoky eyes

1 Prep the eye and powder lightly; this will help with the blending. Apply a smoky chocolate-brown shadow under the eye. Keep the shape slightly rounded (as shown).

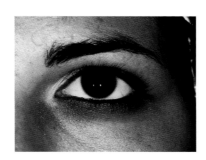

2 Using a large brush, apply a soft wash of the same colour to the whole lid, all the way up to the brow bone, and extend out to the edge of the eye.

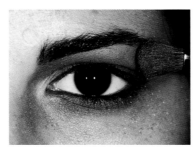

TIP

When you're applying the black pencil to the eye, pull it out and don't let it stop suddenly. Don't let it look too square.

3 Apply a heavy black kohl pencil to the inside rim of the eye and also messily above the whole top lash line, pulling the line out slightly. Heat up the pencil by rubbing it on the back of your hand, and blend the line above the top lashes.

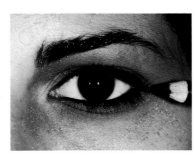

4 Mix black with khaki eye shadow and smudge it around the whole eye, close to the lash line. Use a small rounded brush to blend.

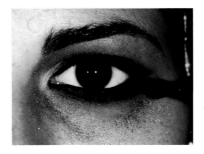

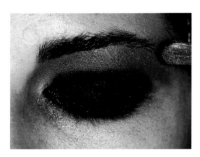

5 Wet the brush, and smudge the black/khaki shadow up towards the brow bone. Don't worry if the line isn't perfect, as you will be blending another colour with it all the way up to the brow bone.

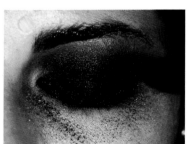

6 Apply an aubergine eye shadow all the way under the brow, blending it to soften the black edges.

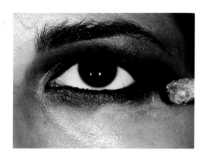

7 Clean up under the eye. Apply your foundation base. Use corn-silk powder to blend the black under the eye. Curl lashes, then apply a full set of false lashes. It is very important to define the brows with this look. Finish with a metallic green shadow in the inner corner of the eye.

LASHES USED

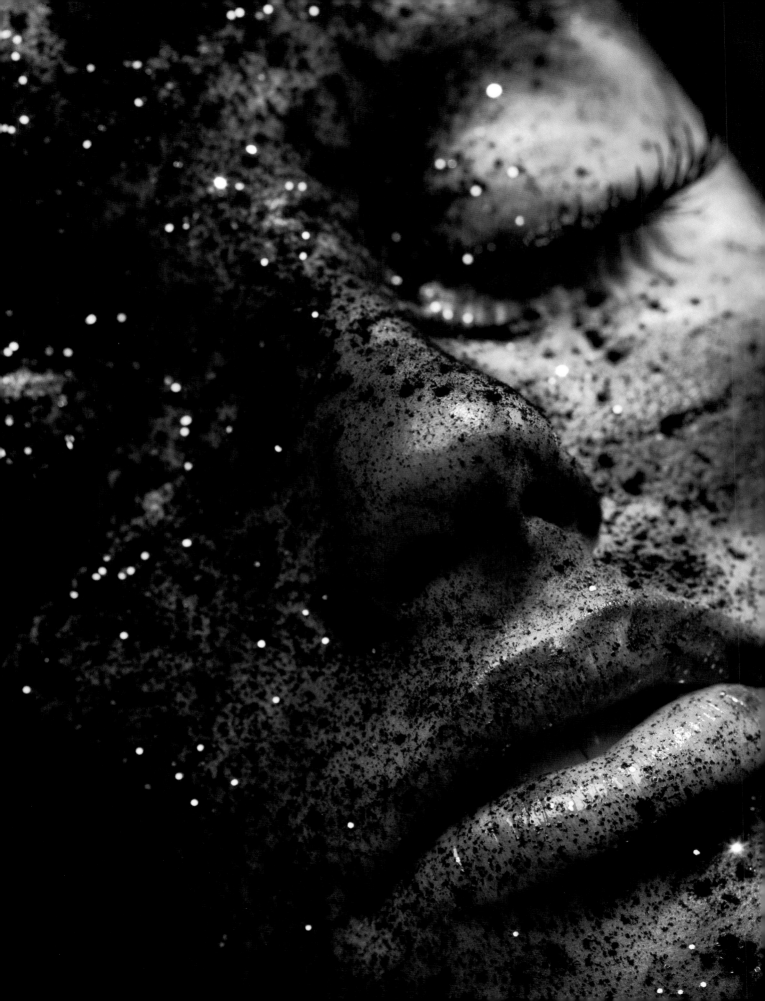

classic eyes

1 Prep the eyes and powder well. Using a large brush, apply a nude matt eye shadow to the whole eyelid.

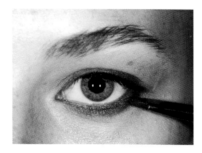

2 Using a thin brush, apply a taupe/oyster-grey shadow to the entire eyelid, and along the bottom lash line.

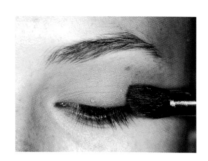

3 Apply a black eyeliner pencil to the inner rim of the eye. Apply the eyeliner heavier in the outer corner V of the eye—you can use a brush as shown.

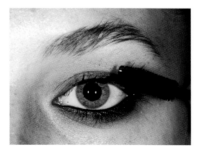

4 Curl lashes, then apply plenty of black mascara to both the top and bottom lashes.

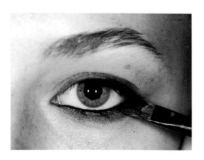

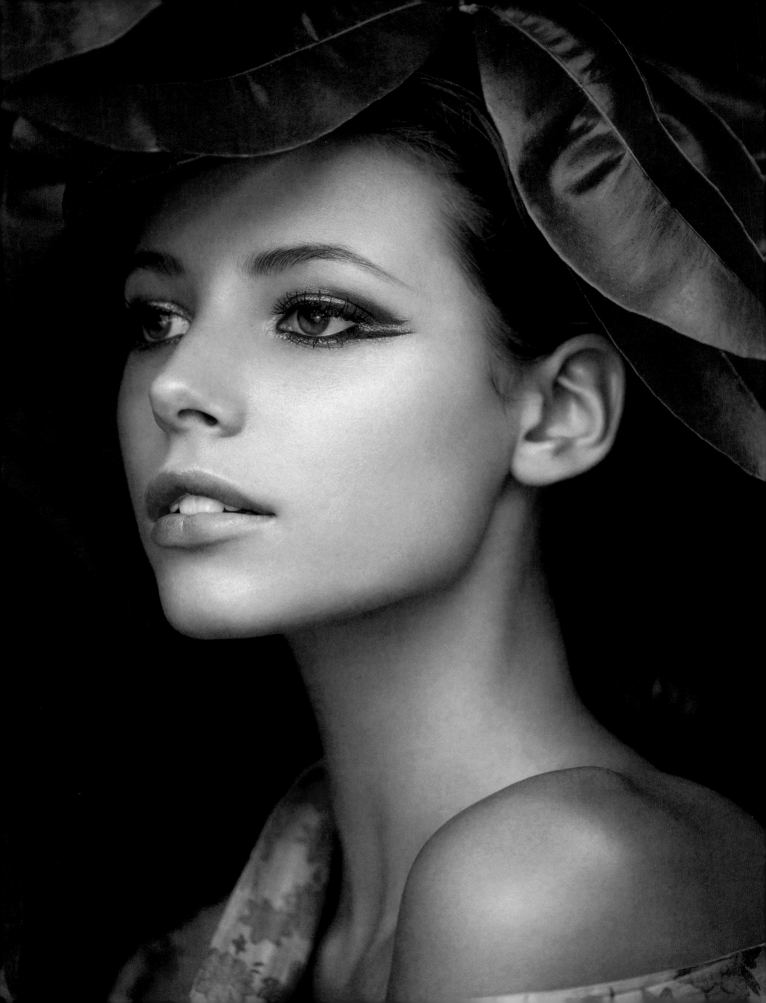

grecian eyes

1 Prep the eyes. Apply black eyeliner heavily to the inner rim of the eye, allowing it to thicken and drop a little as you extend it to the outer corner (as shown). Then, using a small brush, smudge the line and extend out on a slightly upward angle.

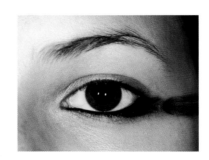

2 Dip a wet thin brush in copper pigment, then apply heavily to the under-lid as shown, keeping it close to the lash line, and stopping two-thirds of the way along.

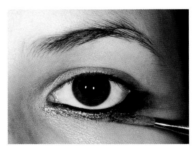

TIPS

The eye shadow should not go above the brow bone for this look.

This is not recommended for small eyes.

3 Wet your brush again, dip it in copper pigment and apply all over the eyelid. Wait for it to dry before you look straight ahead. If you don't want this intensity, you can apply a similar colour in a dry eye shadow.

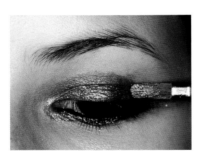

4 Apply black kohl pencil heavily to the outer corner of the eye. Let it sit a minute to allow your skin to heat it up; this makes it much easier to blend.

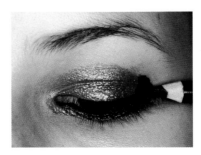

TIPS

If you wish, you can use another colour (instead of the copper) to cut the black in half.

This look is brilliant for rounded or bulging eyes, as the winged effect of the false eyelashes reshapes the eyes.

Be gentle when applying mascara over a false lash; if you use too much pressure, it will rip off. Make sure mascara is the very last thing you do, as having drops of pigment along the lash line can make the eye look dirty and unfinished.

LASHES USED

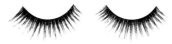

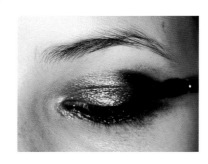

5 Dip a wet brush in black eye shadow, and blend into a V shape (as shown). Yes, this may be difficult, so you will need to practise. This blending is essential as you need to soften the edge. If you're struggling, dip a clean brush in translucent powder to blend the black.

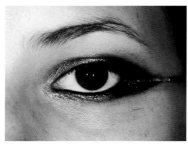

6 Using an eyeliner brush, apply copper pigment to the outer corner of the eye. The idea is to split the black shadow into two lines, as this is a very effective technique, and was used a lot in the 1960s (remember Twiggy?).

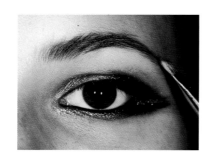

7 Using a brush, define your eyebrows with a soft eye shadow that is the same colour as your brow hair.

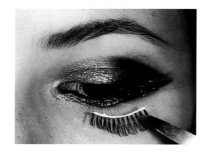

8 Curl lashes, then apply a full set of false lashes that have been cut to create a winged effect. Use eyelash glue to attach the lashes. Wait for it to to thicken before applying. Wait 5 minutes then apply black mascara to the top and bottom lashes.

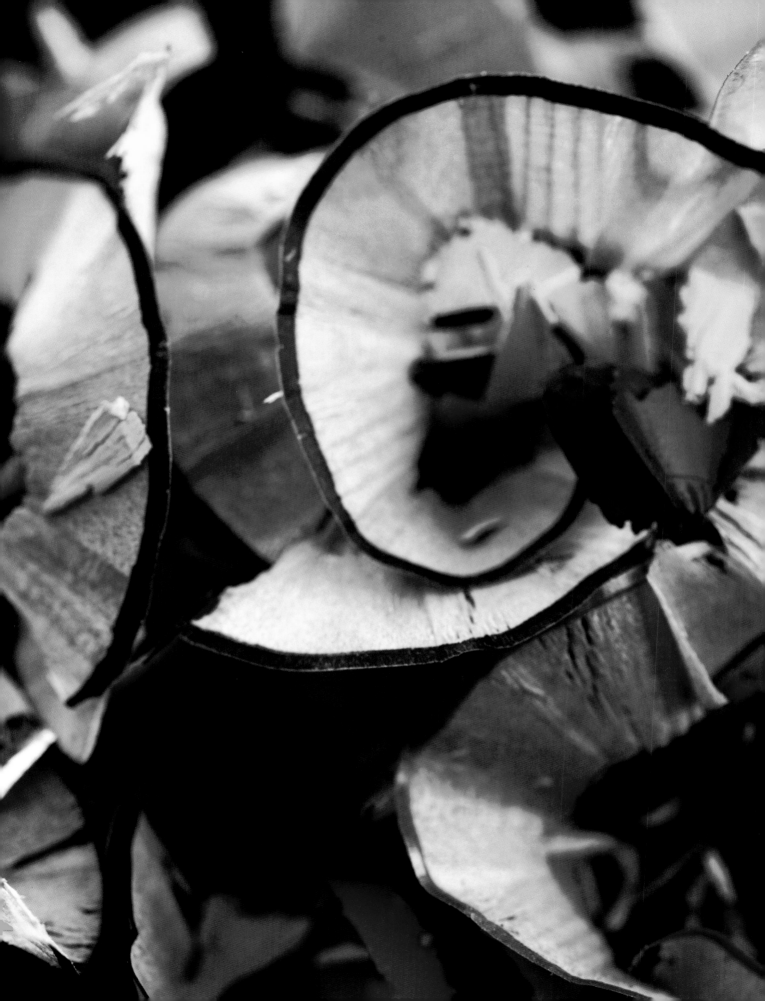

metallic eyes

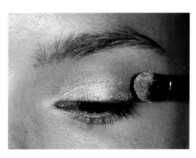

1 Prep the eyes but don't powder. Using a wet medium brush, apply a wash of metallic silver pigment to the whole eyelid. Make sure the application is quite fine, otherwise it will crack with time.

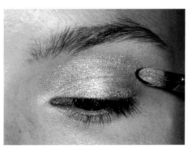

2 Wet the brush again, then apply a diamond dust (or paler shade of silver) to blend the colour higher to just under the brow bone. Also apply an extra amount to the middle of the eyelid. This gives a beautiful highlight.

LASHES USED

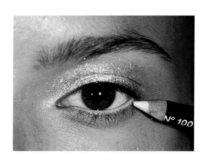

3 Apply an eggshell-white pencil to the inner rim of the eye. Remember, this will fade so you will need to reapply it.

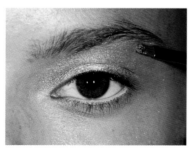

4 Apply a very intense diamond dust all over the eyelid and under the brows. Don't do this on eyes that are a bit puffy, as it will accentuate that puffiness. Finish by applying mascara to your top lashes and then appyling fine false lashes.

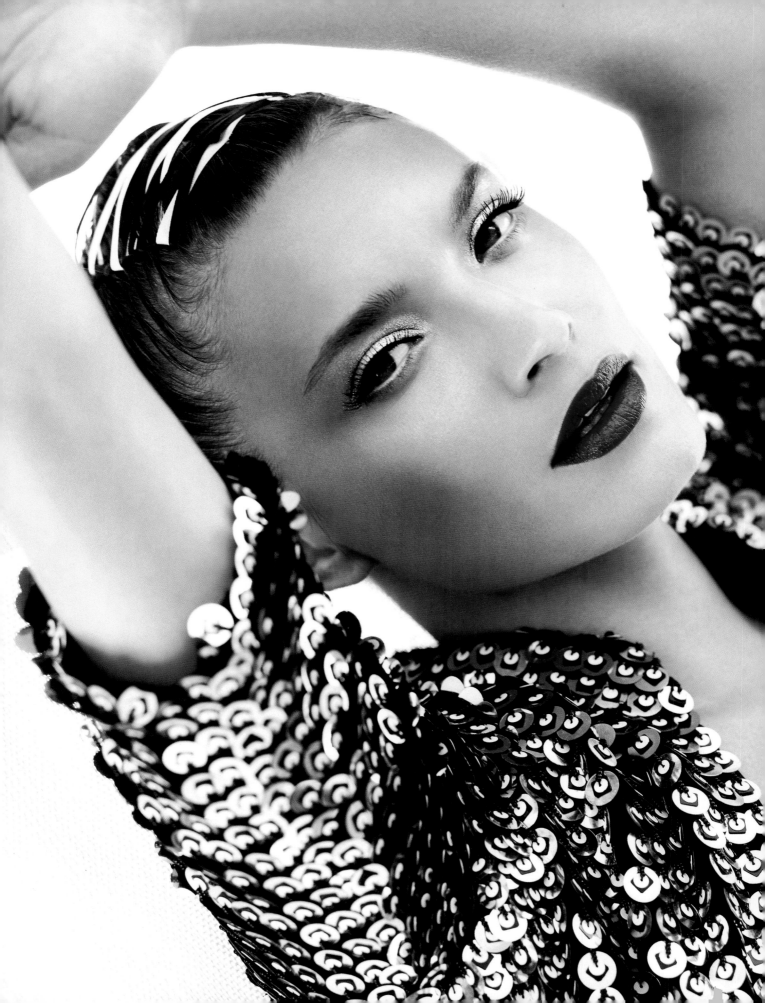

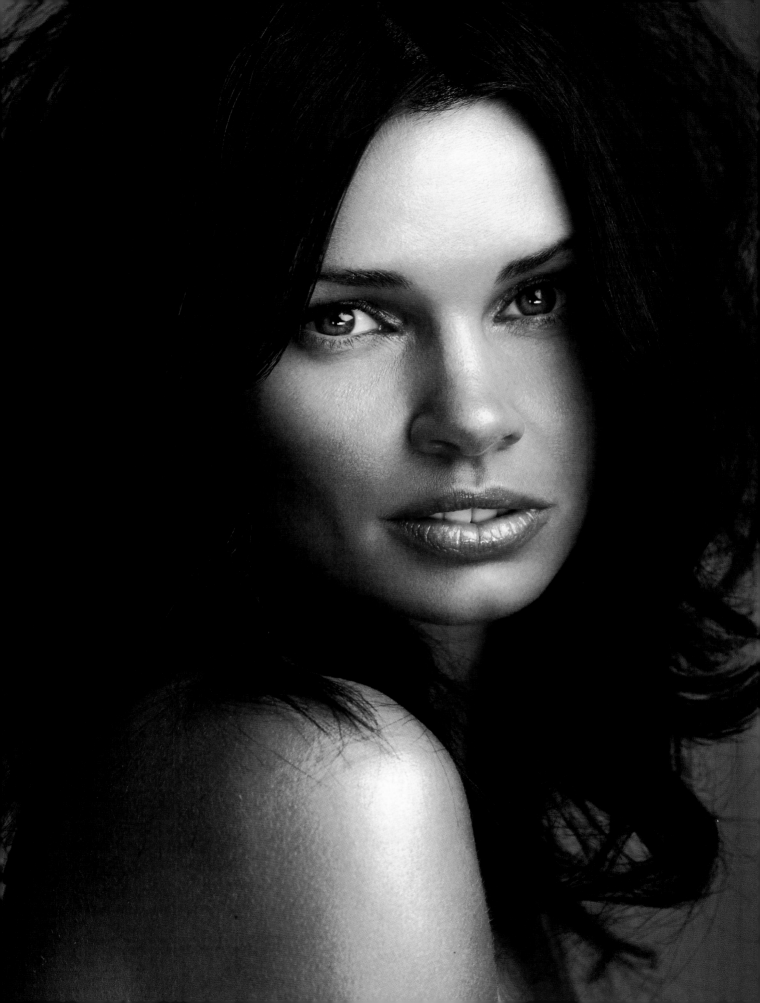

natural eyes

1 Prep the skin but don't powder. Use foundation mixed with illuminiser to give the skin a glowing finish. Then apply a soft gold glitter pigment all over the eyelid (don't go to the brow bone). This gives the illusion of dewy eyes.

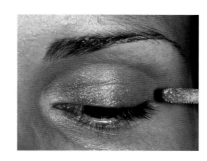

2 With the eyes open, apply an intense amount of glitter to the inner corner. Glitter gels are much better than loose glitter, as they don't get into the eye.

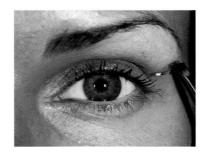

TIP

You don't need to prep the eye with powder for this look. If you need to, you can apply foundation to the eye, but it's not necessary.

3 Clean up and define the brows (see the Eyebrows chapter on page 22). Apply a thin coat of black mascara to the top lashes only. Comb it through when the lashes are still wet to prevent clumping.

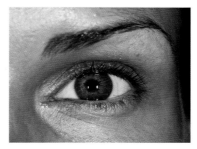

4 Apply single false lashes to the outside of the top lashes. Finish by applying a cheek stain, and a pinky-peach gloss to the lips.

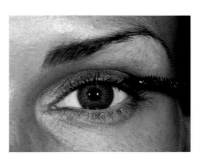

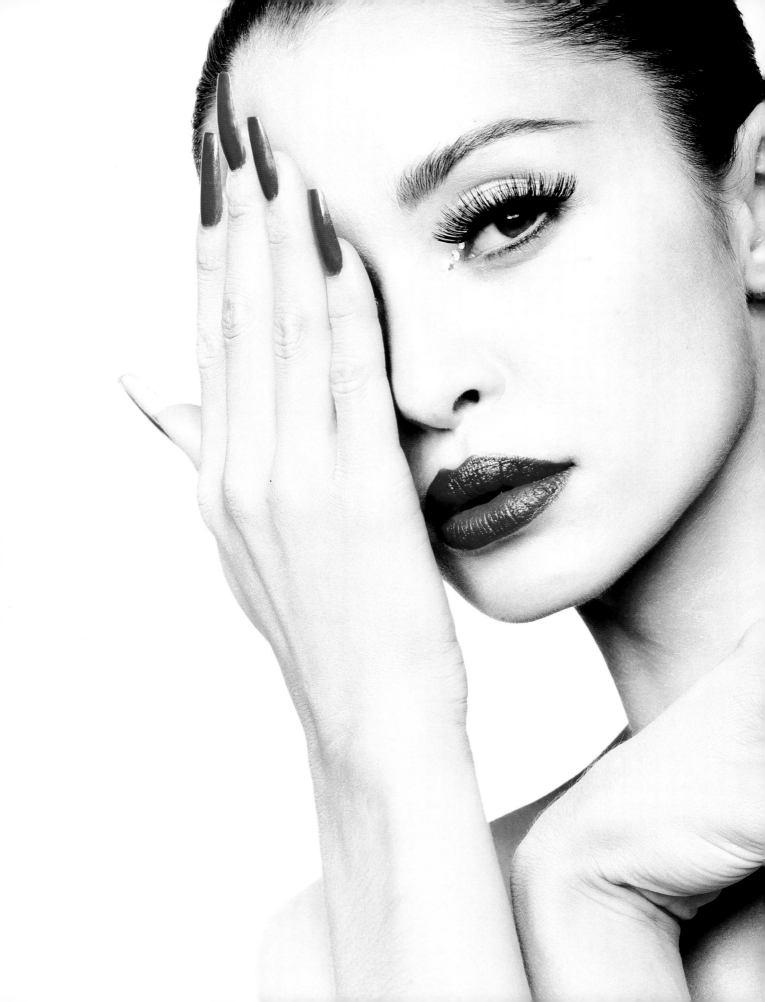

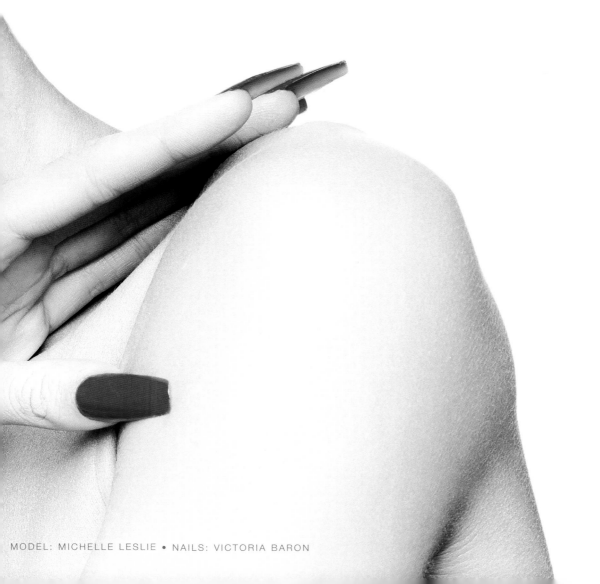

MODEL: MICHELLE LESLIE • NAILS: VICTORIA BARON

asian eye shapes are different to that of Western eyes, so I approach them differently when applying makeup. For example, I always use lengthening mascara and single false lashes because, in most cases, eyelashes are sparse and tend to grow downwards (this is probably why in Asia eyelash curlers can be found more easily than sushi).

I find Asian women's eyes so beautiful to work with because of the shape, which lends itself to a unique style of makeup. This is the eye that is 'made for eyeliner' and bold colour. And in most cases, this eye shape is smaller in size and the main goal is to enlarge it.

Making up Asian eyes is a whole book in itself (which I hope to do one day). I decided to go with looks that are the most sought-after, and those that will work every time.

While I was researching books on Asian eye makeup, I was surprised to see that in most cases the makeup was the same: natural, natural, natural, a bit of eyeliner, lots of mascara, and the only variety given to the lip colour.

Well, Asian women do have the best lips (I personally would die for them), so bold, bright lips are easy to do. And in my experience, nearly every Asian friend or client I have wants bright, colourful and strong, smoky eyes. Asian women love colour; in fact, they love makeup even more than Western women: more makeup is sold in Asian countries than in the whole Western world.

Here are some tips for Asian eyes

- False lashes are your new best friend.
- Only use waterproof eyeliner because your top eye line is mostly hidden when your eyes are open, and it can smudge.
- Own an eyelash curler.
- Consider eyelash extensions.
- Always define your brows.
- Consider lightening your brows because not only does it soften the look, it softens the hair, making brows easier to comb up.
- Eyelash perming, if done correctly, is amazing, but if it's not done in the hands of a pro, your lashes can be burnt off. I've seen serious eye infections and I've seen lashes that do a full 360-degree loop—not recommended.

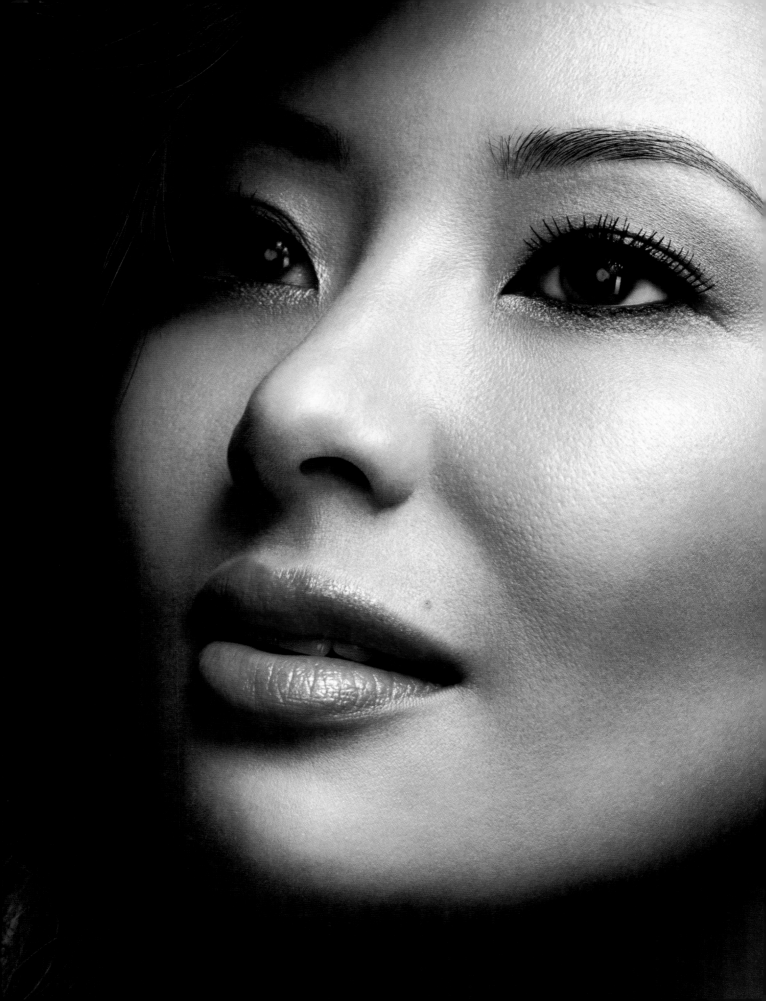

sultry eyes

1 Prep the eyes and powder well. Using a small brush, apply a metallic apricot colour finely just above the eyelid fold.

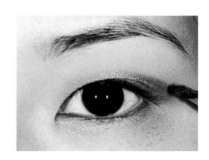

2 Using a wider brush, apply a soft peachy copper shadow and blend above the lid but below the brow, using a circular motion.

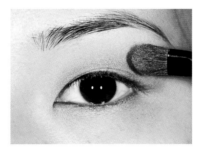

TIP

It's important to enhance the middle of the eyes, to open them up and make them appear wider.

3 Turn the brush upside down, and load it with a deep purple colour. Keep the shape rounded and blend up to the eye fold.

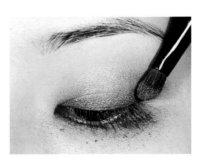

4 Apply an aubergine eyeliner to the inner rim of the eye, extending it out slightly from the lash line.

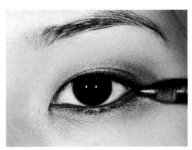

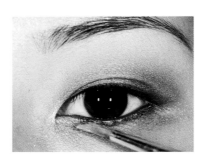

5 Using a fine brush, apply silver to the inner eye, stopping one-third of the way along.

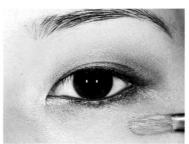

6 Clean up fallout under the eye and apply your foundation.

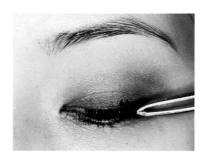

7 Apply short individual lashes, wait for the glue to dry, then apply lots of mascara to the top and bottom lashes.

LASHES USED

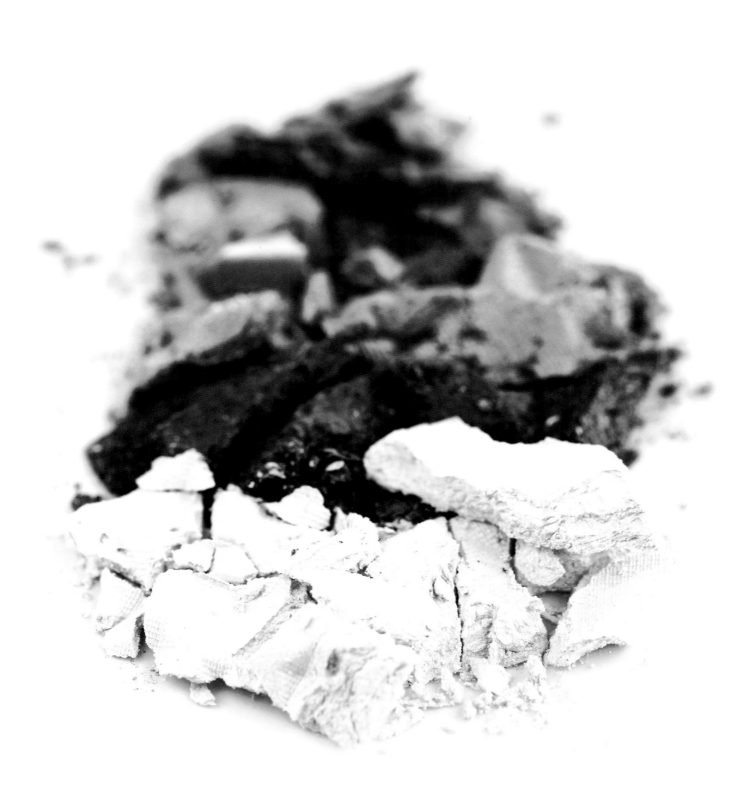

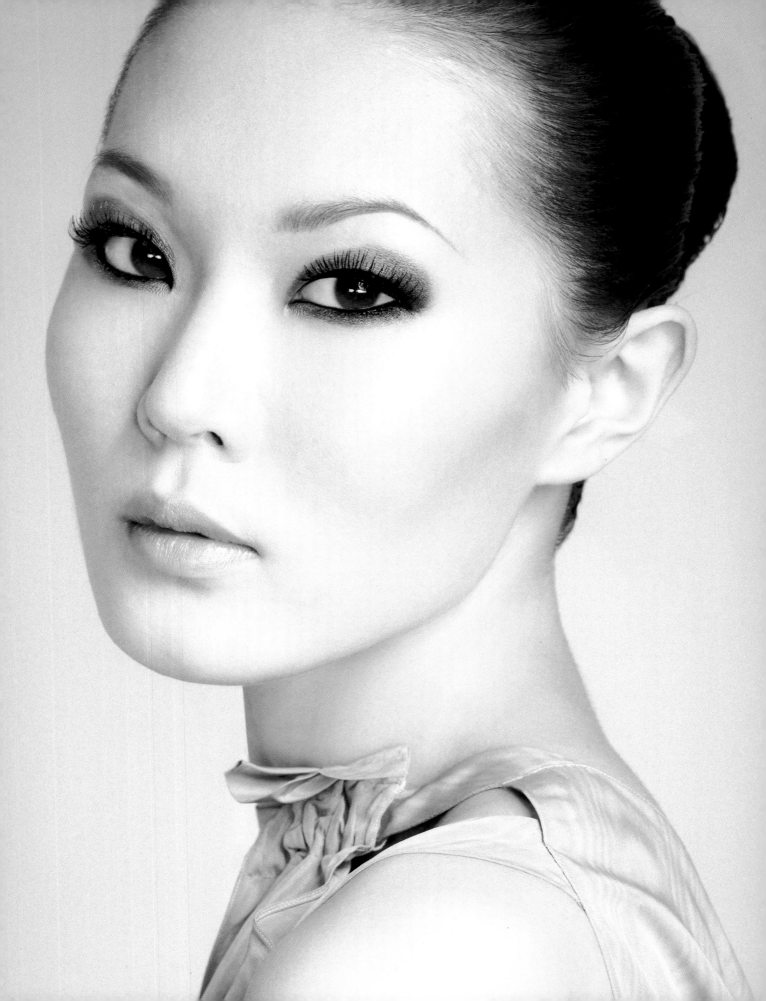

china doll eyes

1 The 'before' shot clearly shows the distance between the brow and eyelid. I want to minimise this distance by doing a smoky eye with a harder edge.

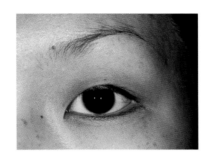

2 Prep the eye and powder well. You'll be using intense eye shadow here, so the more you powder the easier the blending will be.

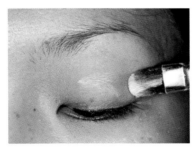

LASHES USED

3 Because of the distance between Xiya's brows and lash line, I want to lower her brow a little. To do this, I have used an eye shadow on her brow (with an angled brush) that is two shades darker than her natural brow colour. Notice that I have gone under her brow line.

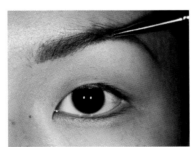

4 Apply a strong wash of violet in a rounded shape to the eyelid as shown, concentrating on the outer eyelid.

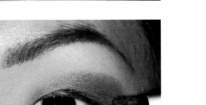

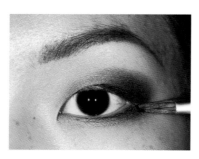

5 Using a small brush, apply violet eyeliner to the outer edge above and below the eye. This will give the colour more intensity and is what enlarges the eye.

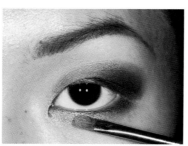

6 Apply a metallic light-blue eye shadow close to the lower lash line, two-thirds of the way along the bottom and one-third along the top lid. Note that I have not blended the edge; this gives the slight illusion of a socket and enlarges the eye.

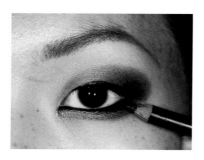

7 Apply an intense black kohl pencil to the inner rim of the eye. As with any application to the inner rim, you will need to reapply throughout the day or evening.

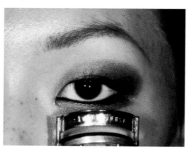

8 Curl your lashes, then apply single false lashes all the way along the top. Wait for the lash glue to dry, then apply two coats of jet-black mascara to both top and bottom lashes. If you have the skill, apply mini single lashes along the bottom lash line as well.

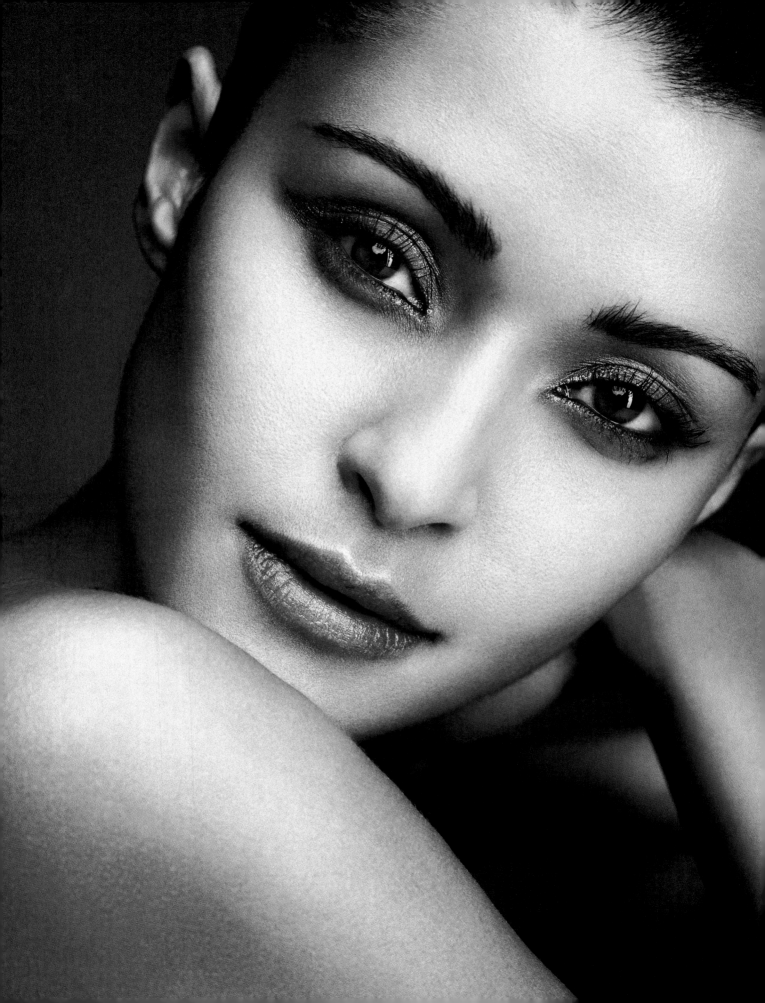

aqua eyes

1 Using a medium brush, apply a mahogany shimmery eye shadow to the whole eyelid, just below the brow bone. Mahogany is one of the best eye shadows you can use as it will go with all eye colours and skin tones.

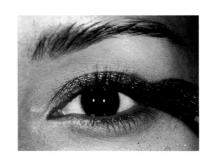

2 Apply an aqua-green eye pencil in the inner rim of the eye. Always remember this will fade as a result of blinking, so you need to reload it. My second choice of colour would be a chocolate bronze.

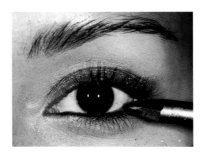

TIPS

Extending the eyeliner as shown in step 4 gives the eye a sleeker look.

Finish the look by applying mascara to the top and bottom lashes.

3 Using a thin brush, apply a teal-blue pigment all around the edge of the eye. A good tip is to wet the brush to make the colour intense and to keep it from running into the mahogany eye shadow.

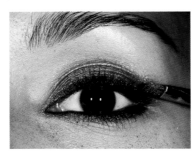

4 Apply a thick layer of black kohl to the outer rim of the eye. Add some aqua glitter eyeliner to the inside top and bottom corners, close to the lash line. Use a black eyeliner pencil and smudge into the outer eyelash line. Then use a brush as shown to extend the line.

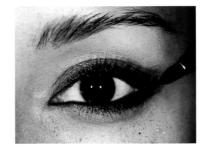

kabuki eyes

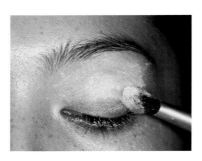

1 Prep the eyelid and apply lots of powder to the area of the eye where you are *not* going to apply eyeliner. Sometimes if the eyeliner is still wet and hits your lid (because you have looked up too quickly) it will mark; this will prevent that and absorb any excess oil.

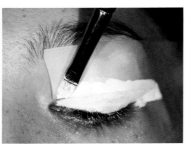

2 With your eye looking straight down, apply tape on a slight tilt. Yes, this is hard to do yourself at home; the best trick is to tilt your head back and look into the mirror. I've used a water-based eyeliner, sweeping across the lid, and extending it out.

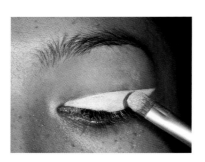

3 Wait until the eyeliner is dry, then set it with white eye shadow (you can skip this step but it helps make it last longer).

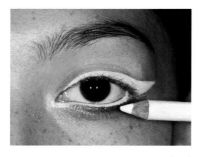

4 Apply white pencil to the inner rim and inner corner of the eye.

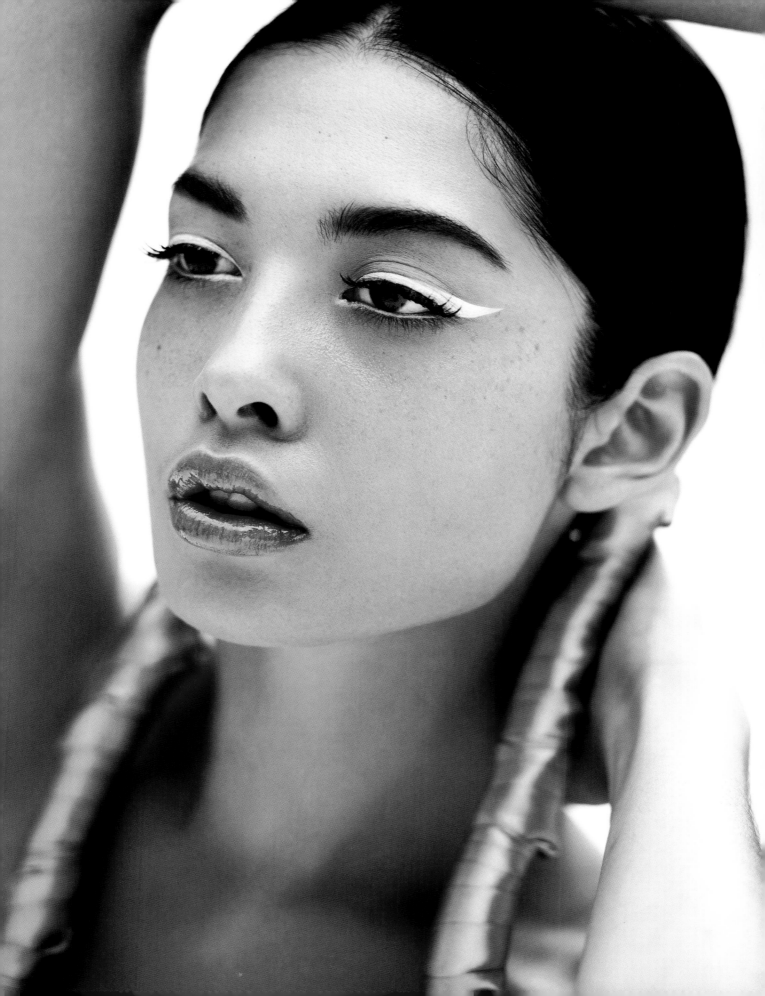

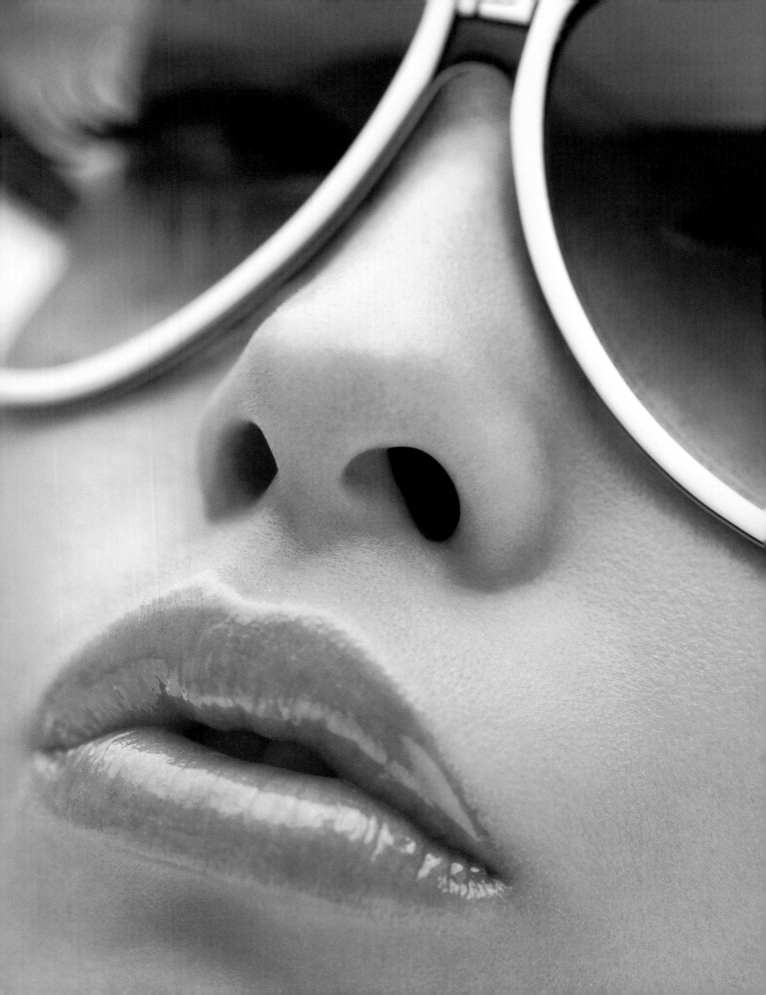

5 Curl lashes then apply mascara to the top lashes only.

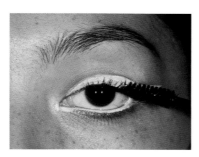

TIP
Remove any white paint you may have in your lash line before applying mascara, as this will make the mascara look grey.

LASHES USED

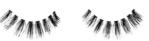

6 Apply a delicate false lash all the way along your lash line (see the False Eyelashes chapter on page 30).

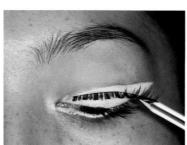

7 Reapply mascara to the top lashes only when the glue has dried.

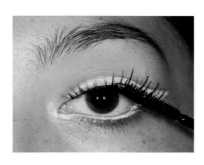

137

over 40s

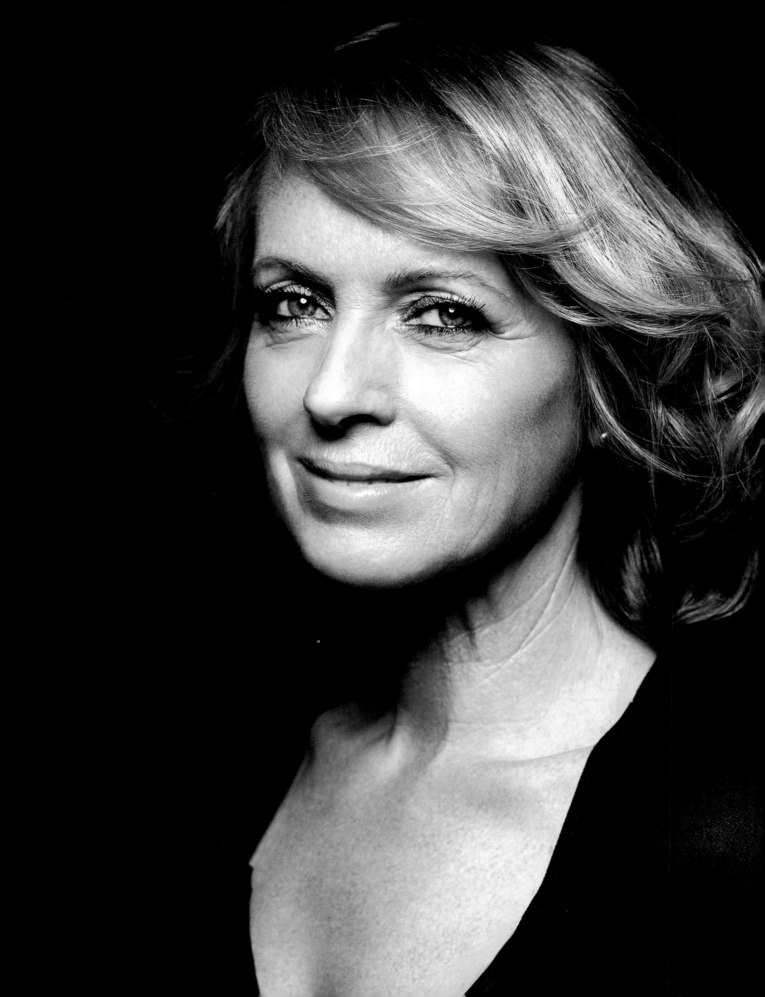

When you are over 40, you shouldn't be wearing the same makeup you wore as a teenager. Not only does it look inappropriate, but as we age so do our facial features and skin tone, making it essential to do makeup differently. Over the years, I've accumulated some indispensable guidelines for women over 40.

Wear more blush

As we age, we lose pigment in the skin, and in most cases the skin has less glow, so you need to step up the blush to restore it.

Never, ever use beige or pink-based foundation

Here is how to age yourself instantly: what most women don't know is that pink, beige or any cool-coloured base powder or foundation sucks warmth out of the skin, something you don't want to do. Anything cool-toned appears paler on the skin than what it actually is (that washed-out look). Have you ever looked back at photos and wondered why your face can be up to two shades paler? This is something the naked eye doesn't always pick up, but the camera does (especially when the flash is on).

Don't over-pluck your brows

Fine eyebrows in the 1940s and 1950s worked—think Marlene Dietrich, or Betty Davis, but unless they are pencilled in precisely, guess what is the best way to age yourself (by at least 10 years)—and why would anyone want to do that? As we age, our eyelids become fuller and droopier, and they begin to sag. If you over-pluck your brows you will accentuate the puffiness, and this will drag your eye shape down. I have explained this in full in the Eyebrows chapter (see pages 24–9). If it is too late for you to regrow your brows for reshaping (because you've plucked them to death), then it's important for you to learn how to fill them in (see the Eyebrows chapter).

Don't use more eyeliner under the eye than on top

Please do this exercise for me: stand in front of the mirror, take both your pointer fingers and place them directly in the middle of your lower eyelids—right in the middle. Now, pull your eyelids down. Not attractive, is it? Well, this is exactly what you're doing when you apply heavy eyeliner or pencil all the way along the bottom lash line, or when your bottom eyeliner is a lot more prominent than the top (it only works on Asian eyes). Here's a great tip: if you are using any eyeliner at all, always make sure that your top line, whether it's eye shadow or pencil, is two to three times heavier than underneath, as this will automatically lift your eyes.

Don't use frosty eye shadow or white frosty highlighter

If you own any, throw it out immediately. Any frosty or shimmery eye shadow or highlighter accentuates lines because it makes the skin look scaly. Also, frosty blues, pinks and purples are designed for teenagers—think Spice Girls here. You don't want to look like that—really.

Don't forget your décolletage—the biggest sign of ageing

There is nothing more unattractive than seeing a well-groomed woman with beautiful makeup that stops at the neck. Yes, our chest area has copped a lot of sun throughout our lives and is one of the major areas that has burst capillaries and pigmentation (if you're prone to it). You would never see an actress or celeb strolling down the red carpet with a bright red neck. So if you go to such efforts to conceal signs of ageing on your face, you should dedicate the same, if not more, effort to your décolletage. It takes no time to apply a soft wash of foundation. This is one area where I love to use mineral makeup. Not only is the powdery texture less likely to rub off on your clothes, most, if not all, contain sunscreen.

Don't over-powder

Unfortunately, the more moisturisers, anti-ageing creams and oils you load up your skin with prior to applying your makeup, the more porous your skin becomes when you use powder. Remember that even the finest powders can look cakey if the skin is too moist and greasy just before application.

Don't use dark or harsh lipstick shades if you have small lips

As we age, our lips begin to sag downwards, so applying harsh liner or dark shades just brings more attention to this. Don't get me wrong—I love seeing women over 40 using bright shades, but you shouldn't make your lips one flat colour. Always highlight the middle of your lips to give them a more rounded, fuller shape. And don't always follow your exact lip line. Use a little concealer or foundation on the outer corners of your mouth, and just go on the inside of your natural lip line on your bottom outer lip corner to help lift your mouth.

Don't overuse lip gloss

Lip gloss makes any lipstick susceptible to running, and if you have lines around your lips, whether subtle or deep, gloss will basically turn your lipstick into soup and make it bleed. I am always asked how to stop lips from bleeding, and my number one response is don't overuse gloss; in other words, don't use it all over your lips, just keep it to the centre. Make sure you rub foundation or concealer around (not on) your lips, then powder your face (but not the lips), before applying lipstick and gloss. And in all honesty, most celebs I work with have some sort of temporary or permanent filler (such as restylane or collagen) to fill those small lines. If done well, pumping up your lips ever so slightly can take years off!

And please, please look at using different options for facial hair removal

I know that it's not fun—all of a sudden, we get hairs growing where we never thought possible. And the fine lip and chin hairs we had through our late 20s and early 30s now look and feel like tree stumps. Vow never, ever to go anywhere without tweezers, and to always do a safety check in the rear-view mirror of your car before going anywhere in public. I keep a pair of tweezers in my arm rest because the car mirror has good lighting in the daytime. I also recommend those hideous magnifying mirrors you see in hotel bathrooms. I don't know why they do it to us—hotel rooms should equal holidays and luxury, not frightening new discoveries, down lights and bathroom scales. (If you don't weigh yourself at home, why would some crazy hotel decorator think you would want to do it on holidays?) But at least these mirrors are good for something!

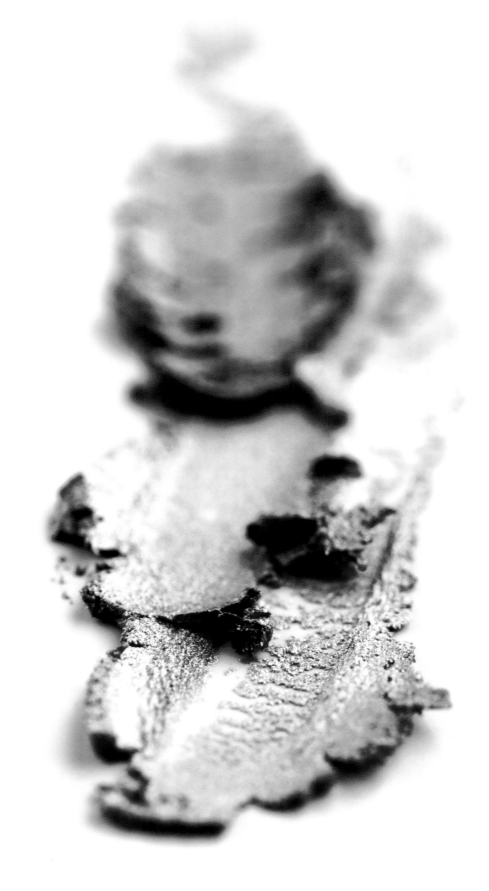

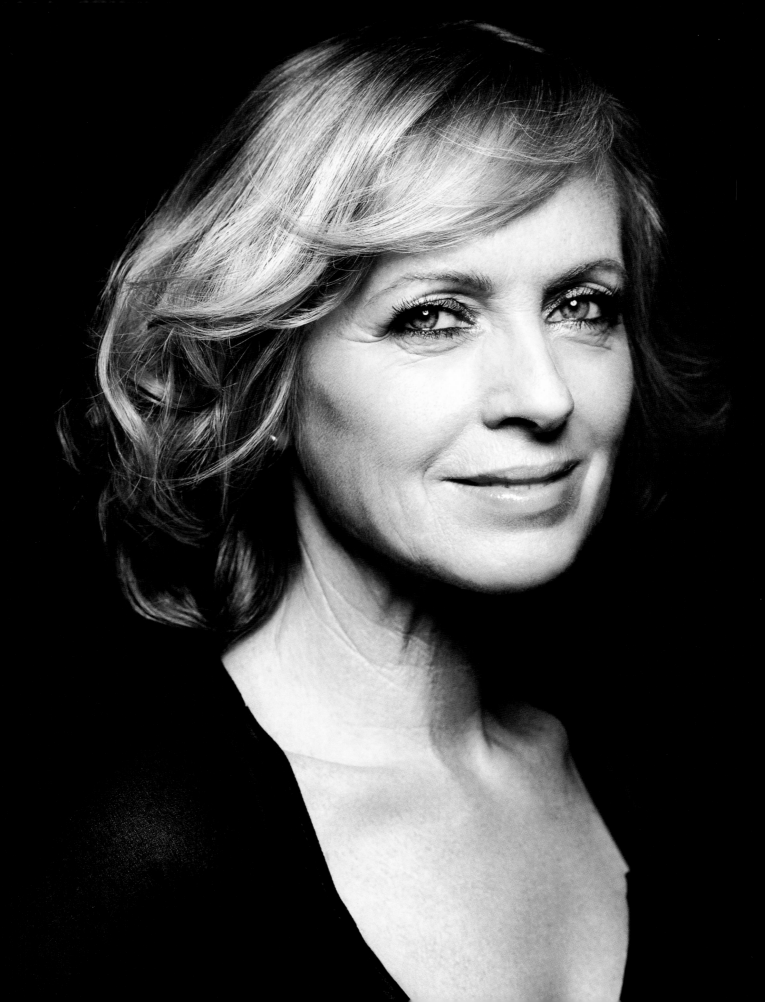

sarah

1 Ensure eyes are prepped well. Using a medium brush, apply a strong wash of high-sheen mahogany eye shadow. Don't cover the entire eyelid, and keep the shape rectangular, not rounded, as a rounded shape can age the eye.

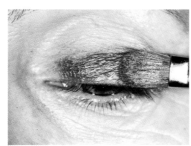

2 Blend the eye shadow by using a fine translucent powder and a small brush. Powder will stop your eye shadow from running and give you a beautifully smooth finish.

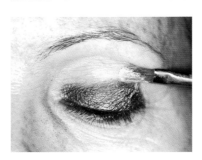

3 Apply a rich black eye shadow to the outer corner of the eye. Don't worry about fallout on the cheeks—this is why I always do the eyes first. If you're having trouble blending, use a clean brush with translucent powder, as this will help soften the edge.

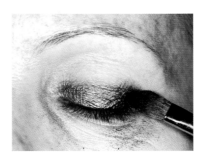

4 Using a wet, extremely fine brush, apply a really golden bronze to the inner corner V shape of the eye. The brush is wet to intensify the colour and prevent fallout, as the fallout will accentuate any wrinkles in this area. The golden bronze colour will make green eyes stand out.

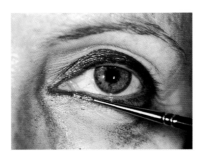

TIPS

When applying eye shadow to mature eyes, always use gentle pressure, as too much pressure will move the skin and cause eye shadow to end up in the wrong place.

The myth is that women over 30 should not wear shimmer or glitter. Notice I am putting it on the inside rim of the eye. That's where it does not move.

I have lightened Sarah's eyebrows with eyebrow mascara.

145

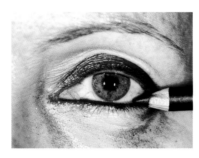

5 Apply a dark chocolate-brown eyeliner heavily to the inner rim of the eye with a non-waterproof pencil. Make sure the pencil is not too sharp. Also, smudge it into the lash line so there are no skin-coloured spaces. If your eyes are small, don't apply to the inner rim.

TIP

For small eyes, use a creamy white pencil in the inner rim instead of the chocolate-brown pencil. This will open up the eyes and make them look bigger and brighter. Keep the chocolate pencil for the eyelash line instead.

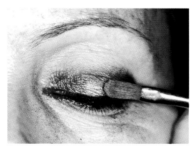

6 Apply a soft gold eye shadow to the centre of the eyelid. This will make the eyes look more alive.

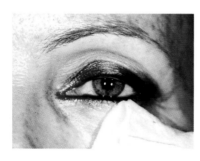

7 Clean fallout from under the eye. Sorbolene cream is terrific for this (remember to be gentle).

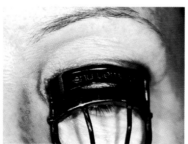

8 Curl eyelashes. Apply black mascara to both top and bottom lashes. Finish by applying single false lashes to the top outer edge of the eye.

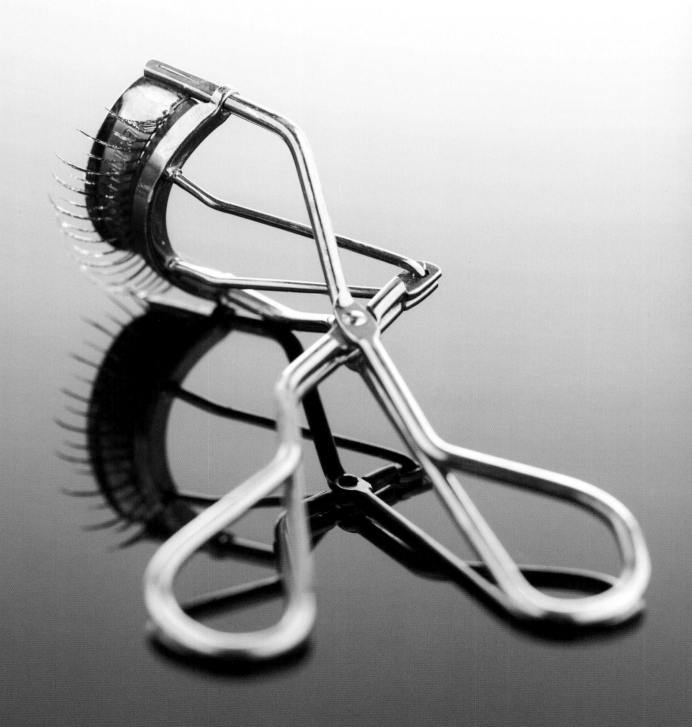

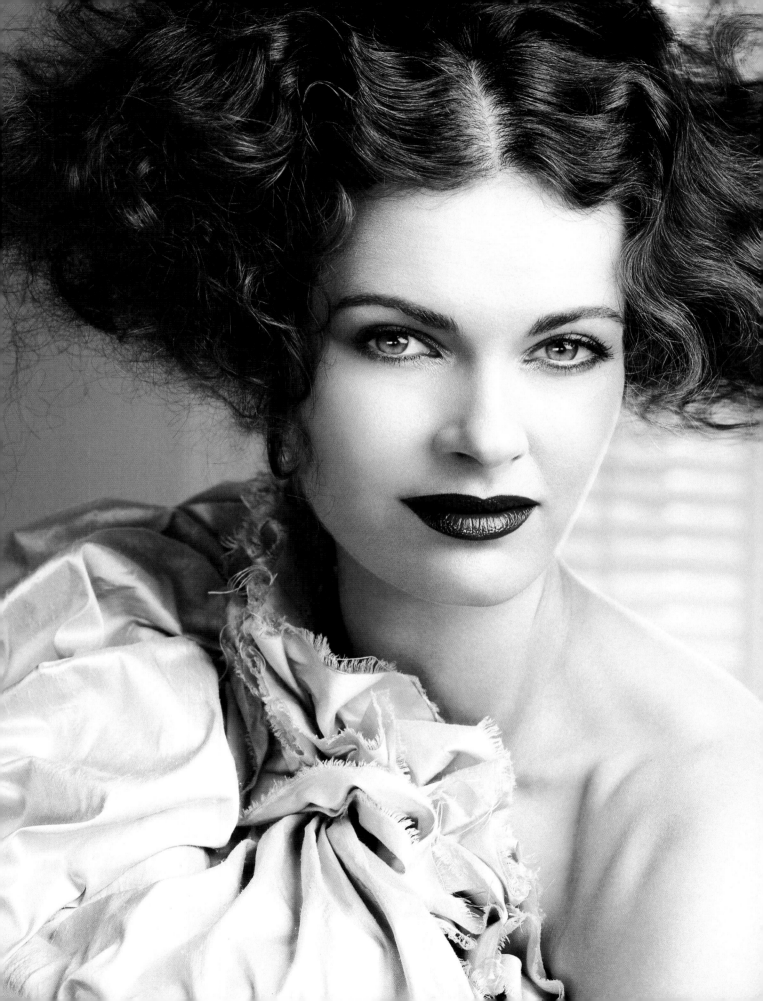

florence

1 Prep eyes and powder well. Using a small brush, apply a soft khaki-gold wash over the lid, emphasising colour on the outer corner. If you are having trouble blending, use a clean brush with corn-silk powder to help blend.

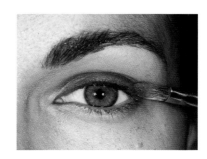

2 Apply a creamy white concealer pencil heavily to the inner rim of the eye. This helps open up the eyes, and makes them look brighter and whiter.

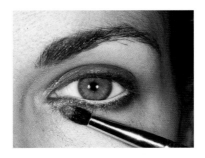

TIP

Have a clean mascara wand on standby to comb through lashes when mascara is still wet.

3 Apply a creamy antique khaki-gold pencil along the lower lash line. Note that I have dropped the line and smudged the pencil down at the outer corner of the eye. This opens up the eye, making it appear larger.

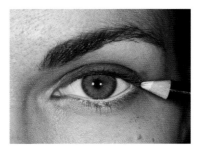

4 Apply a bronze shimmery eye shadow to the inner corner V of the eye. Then, taking the same pencil you used under the eye, apply along the top lash line one-third of the way across the eyelid. Curl lashes and coat with plenty of rich black mascara on both top and bottom.

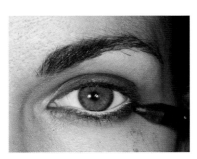

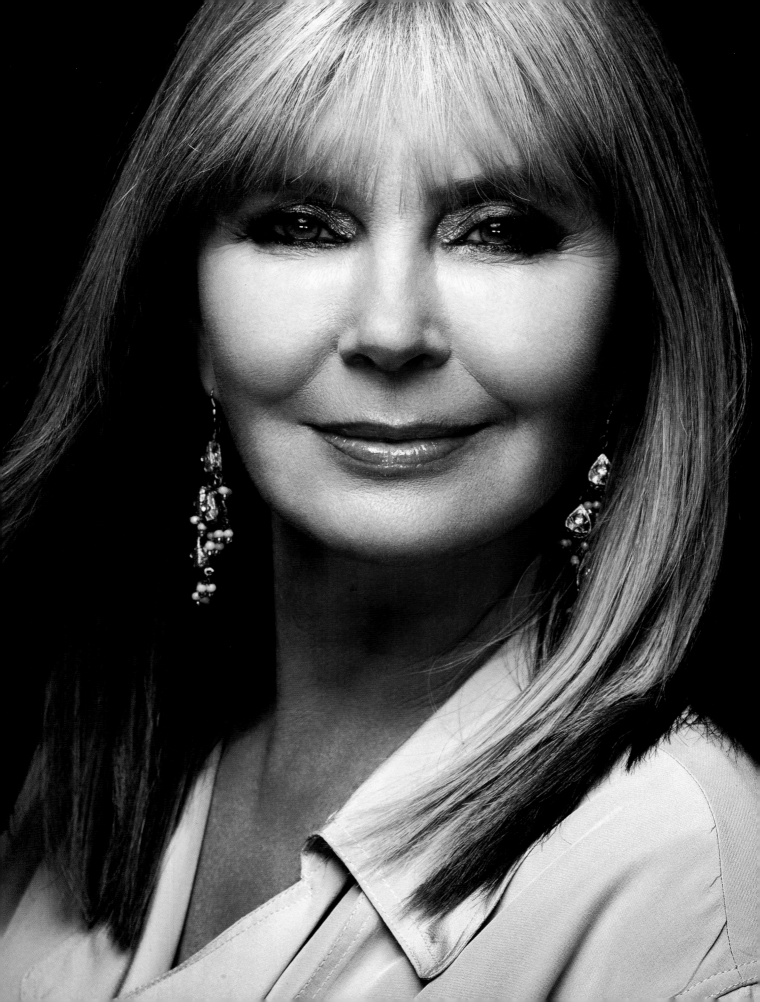

ursula

1 Begin by prepping the eyes well. Using a very fine brush, apply a copper pigment to the inner corner of the eye. Then apply a chocolate-brown pencil heavily to the inner rim of the eye.

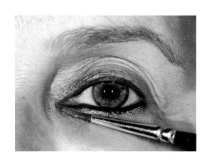

2 Apply a matt chocolate eye shadow to the outer third of the lid, top and bottom. Keep it close to the lash line, extending out only slightly.

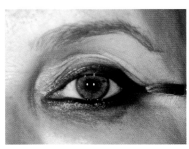

TIPS

Because Ursula has blue eyes, I am working with gold and bronze tones, which make the blue pop out.

The reason you don't want to apply the flesh-gold pigment all the way across the mahogany is that you want to have the depth to make the eye stand out. Also, too much shimmer is tacky.

3 Apply sheer translucent powder to the lid for easier blending, then apply a mahogany-brown pigment to the outer edge of the socket (as shown). Blend across the lid and under the brow bone.

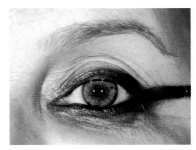

4 Apply a flesh-gold pigment to the open area of the eye and middle of the eyelid. Don't apply all the way across over the mahogany pigment. Finish by applying black eyeliner to the inner rim of the eye and close to the lash line. Apply mascara to top and bottom lashes.

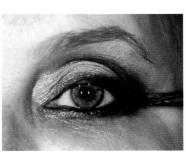

sarah

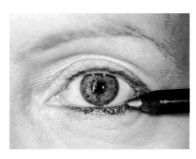

1 I have applied the foundation first here, to show that you can do your foundation before your eyes. This will still allow drops of eye shadow to fall on your cheeks, but you can clean it up afterwards. After foundation, apply a gold eyeliner to the inner rim of the eye.

TIP

It is really important to keep away from eye cream when applying eye shadow. Your eyelids are very oily, and using cream before eye shadow will just make it grab the shadow unevenly.

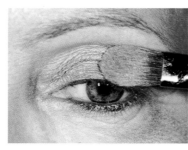

2 Using a large brush, apply an antique, highly pigmented gold shadow to the whole lid to just beneath the brow bone.

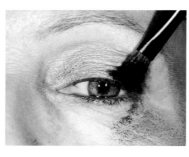

3 Tipping the brush upside down, apply a high-intensity black eye shadow to the outer edge of the upper eyelid. Tipping the brush keeps the intensity along the lash line. Blend out lightly.

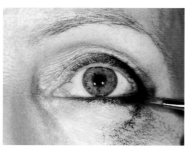

4 Using a small brush, look upwards and apply lots of black eye shadow under the eye as shown. You must keep it close to the lash line and only one-third of the way along. Blend out lightly.

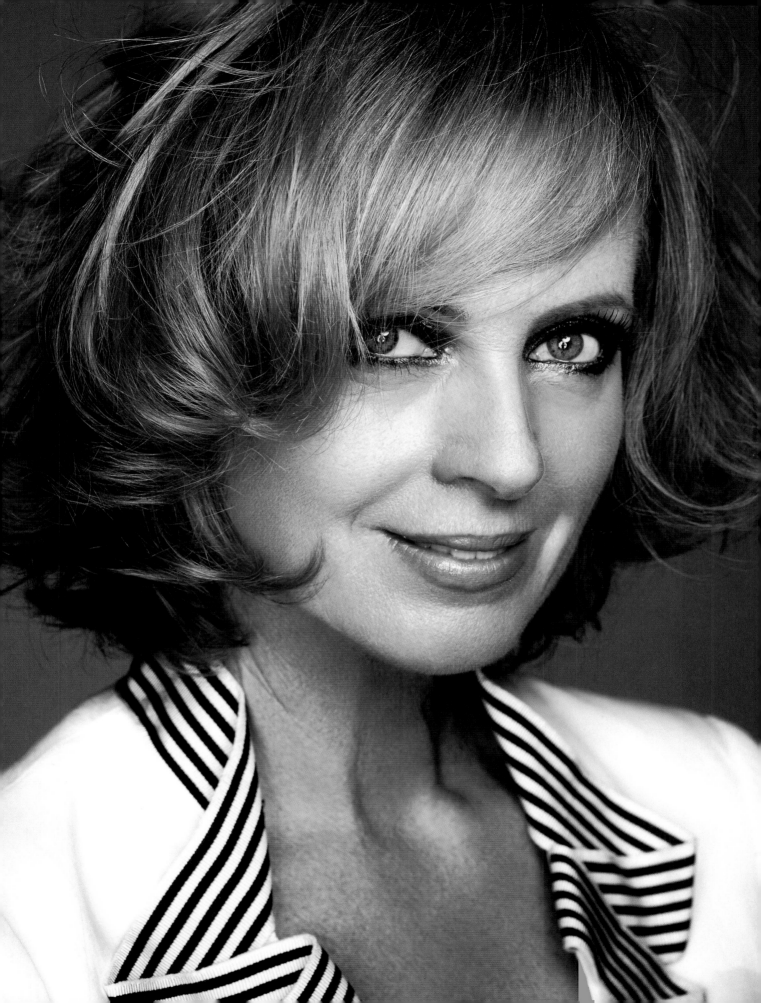

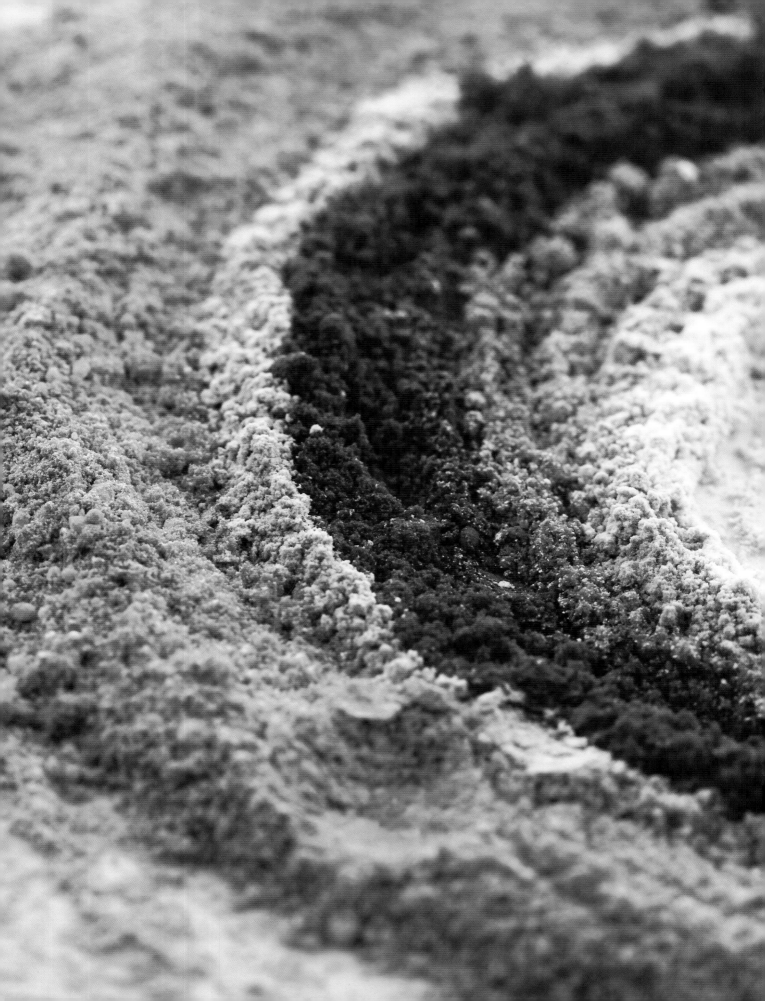

5 Add black eye shadow with a small brush to the top inner eye socket. This way, you create the illusion of a larger eye as it makes the eye shape more rounded and really opens up the area.

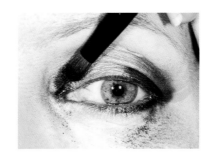

6 Using a smaller brush, apply gold again to blend with the black on the upper lid. A bigger brush will mix too much into the black and it will just get messy.

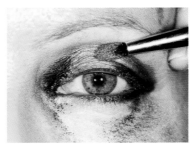

TIPS

It is important to apply the mascara last, otherwise you will get gold fallout on the lashes.

Using a lipstick that is similar to your natural lip tone makes the lips appear larger, as it makes it harder to define the lines of the lips.

7 Wipe up all of the fallout, then reapply foundation to where you have cleaned up the drops of eye shadow. I have added illuminiser to the foundation for a beautiful sheen. This is something women over 40 are told to keep away from. But you can use it and here's the proof.

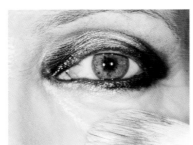

8 To finish off, apply a high-intensity gold pencil to the inside corner of the eye. This opens the eye and makes it more alive. Apply black mascara to the top and bottom lashes. Use a light lipstick similar to your natural lip tone.

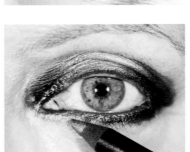

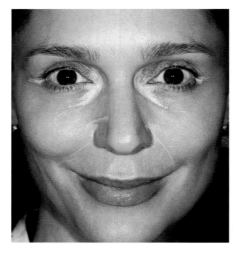

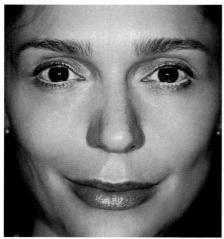

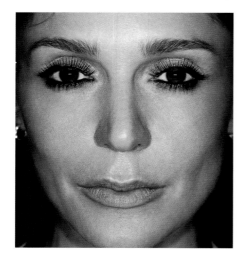

tottie

1 I have applied a light foundation. Because I am going for more of a velvety look on her skin, so that it's not too shiny, I am not using an illuminiser. It is important not to use ten different moisturisers before applying your foundation, as it will cause the foundation to slide, and your eye shadow to crease within seconds of applying.

2 Looking down to stretch out the creases in the lids, apply translucent powder to the face as well as the lids.

3 Using a fine brush, apply antique gold liquid eyeliner along the top lash line, and curl lashes.

4 Apply a full set of natural brown false lashes. Comb brows. Apply bronzer to the cheeks, and blend up to the brow. Remember not to smile while applying the bronzer.

5 Apply black kohl pencil to the inner rim and top outer edge of the eyelid and smudge lightly. Then apply a coat of black mascara to the top and bottom lashes, and a dark bronze eyeliner to the inside of the eye.

6 Then finish by applying a nude lipstick.

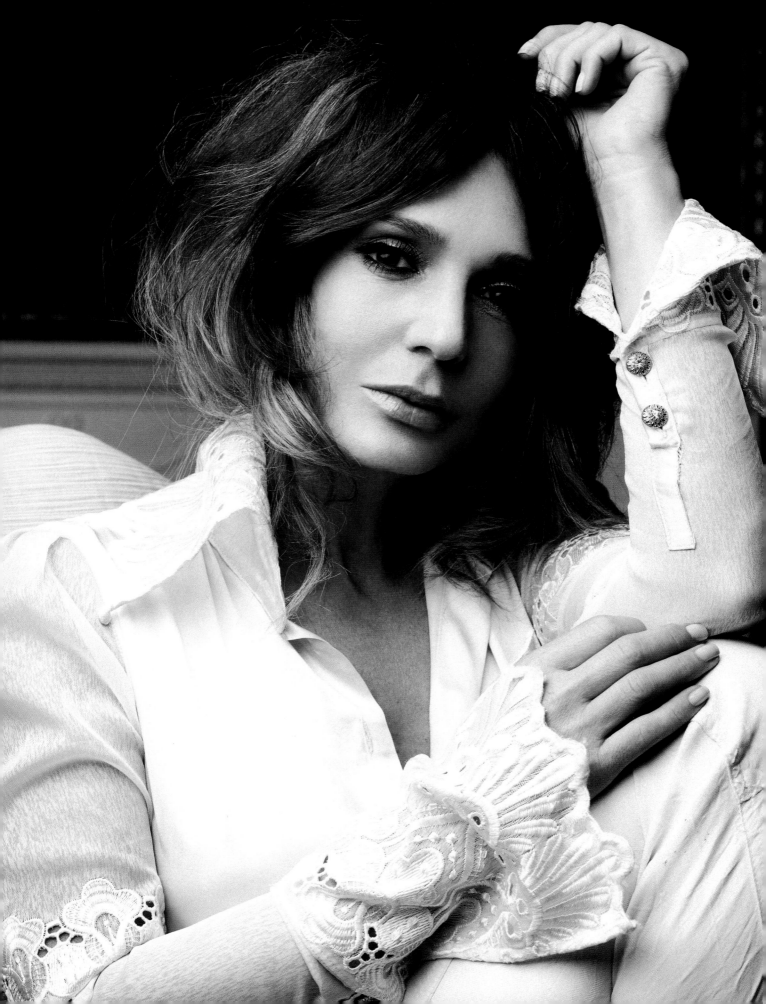

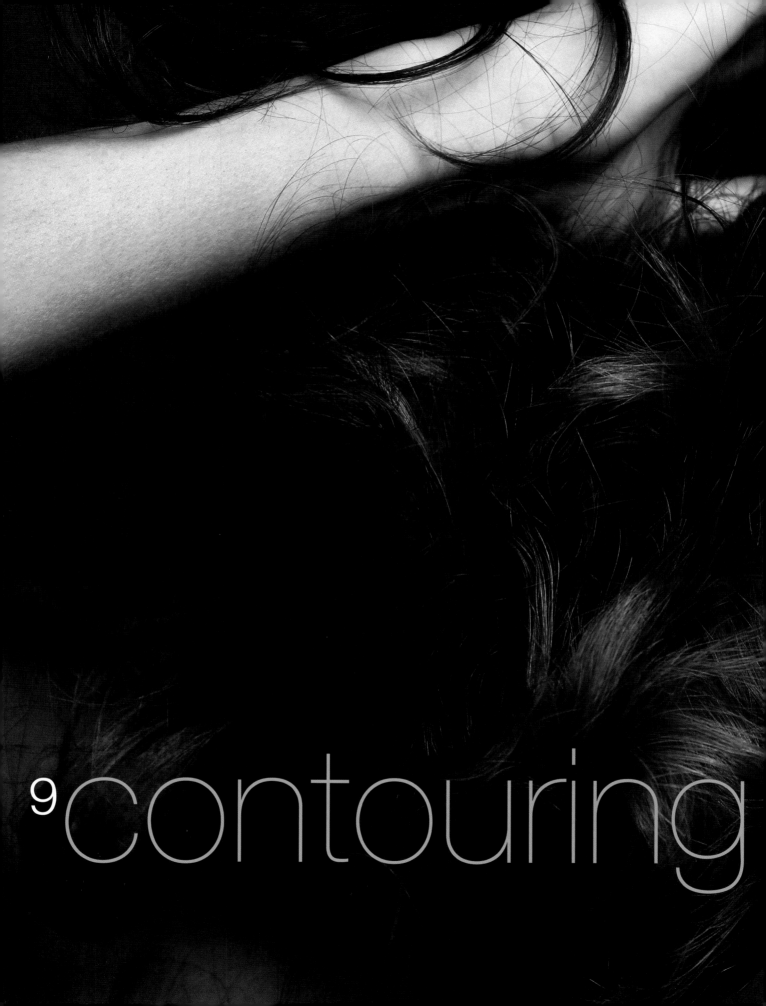

9 contouring

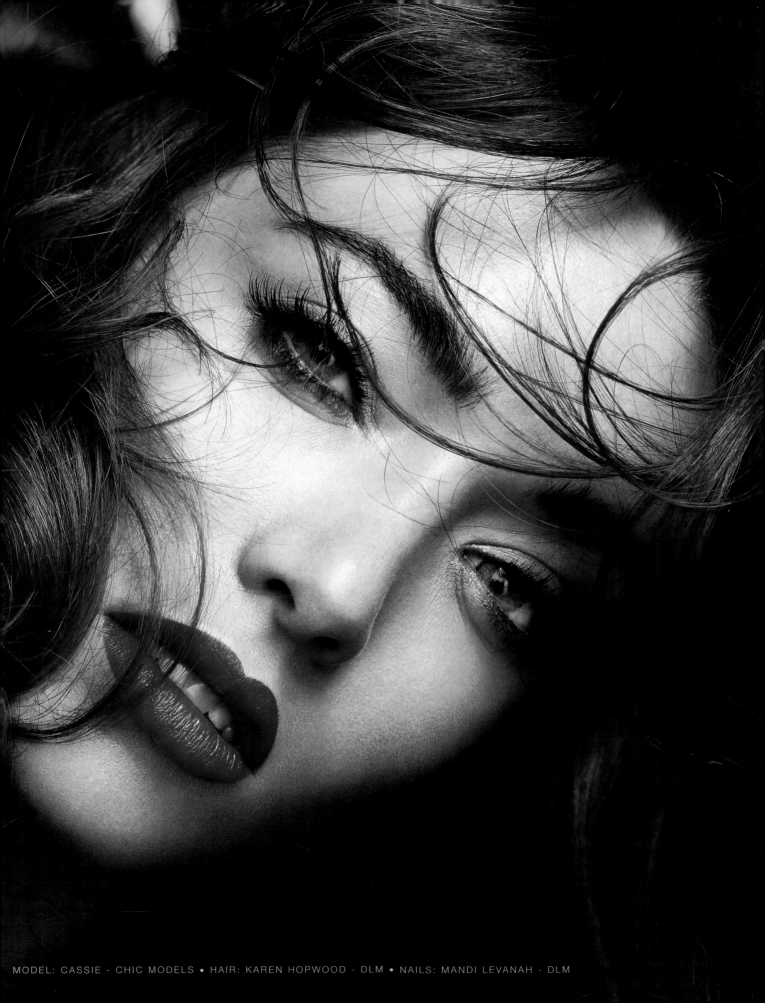

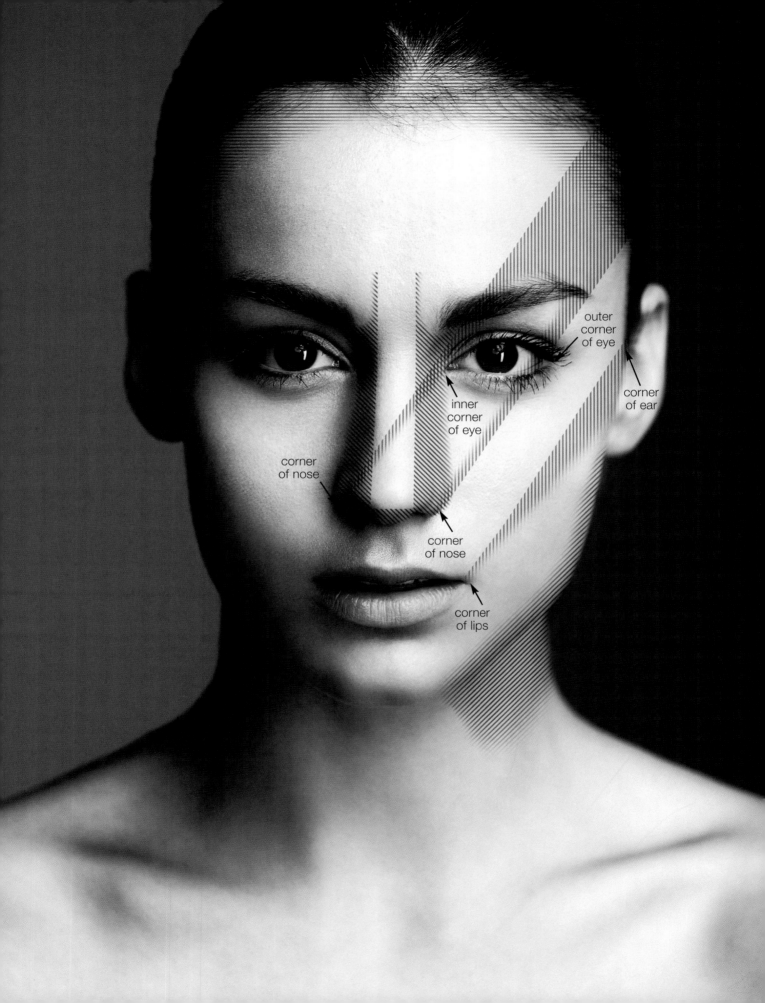

outer
corner
of eye

corner
of ear

inner
corner
of eye

corner
of nose

corner
of nose

corner
of lips

contouring face map

Warning: handle with care! You must check your profile upon completion. Contouring for me means to change, accentuate, hide, strengthen, and define your whole face. The ability to contour is a makeup artist's most powerful weapon. It's also the oldest technique in makeup, one which all the masters still hold as the 'secret tool'. I believe it is contouring that sets apart good makeup artists from the great masters.

However, contouring can seem the most confusing, overwhelming and misleading of techniques. This is one area where if you can't get it right, it's best not to even try. The products to use for contouring are: nude skin-toned blushes and grease- or cream-based foundations two or three shades darker than your natural skin tone.

Why do we contour?
- To give defined cheekbones (no, pink stripes down the side of your face won't achieve it).
- To narrow a larger, or wider, shaped nose.
- To create fuller lips.
- To create a defined jawline.
- To lift sagging eyes.
- To hide a receding hairline.
- To minimise a large forehead.
- To enlarge eyes.

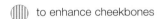 to enhance cheekbones

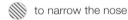 to narrow the nose

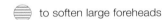 to soften large foreheads

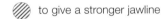 to give a stronger jawline

To take you through this in the simplest of ways, I have taken our model Lizzy B, photographed her with not a scrap of makeup on bar a hint of mascara, and then contoured her step by step by using a cream foundation colour that is four shades deeper than her natural skin tone.

Remember, this technique is advanced. Not many women know about it and not many makeup artists (of the younger generation) use it.

The never, evers
- Never use a shimmery product of any kind for contouring.
- Never use a contouring product that's not a natural skin tone, and it must be at least two to three shades darker than your skin tone.

step 1: shaded cheekbones

Imagine drawing a line from your lip corner to the top of the ear, as shown here. You only shade under this line as contouring pushes features back, therefore lifting your cheekbone. Always start from the ear and blend forwards. Do not start from your cheekbone and work to the ear (as you do with blush) because it's important that darkest part is at your ear and not in the middle of your cheek, or you'll look like you have a bad bruise.

The second imaginary line is from both outer corners of the nose to both outer corners of the eyes. You'll find that these lines will be parallel in nearly every case. You shade in between these lines and not outside, and make sure you blend the edges. This also indents the temple, making the cheeks look more prominent, and it lifts the eyes. This one is my favourite as it takes years off.

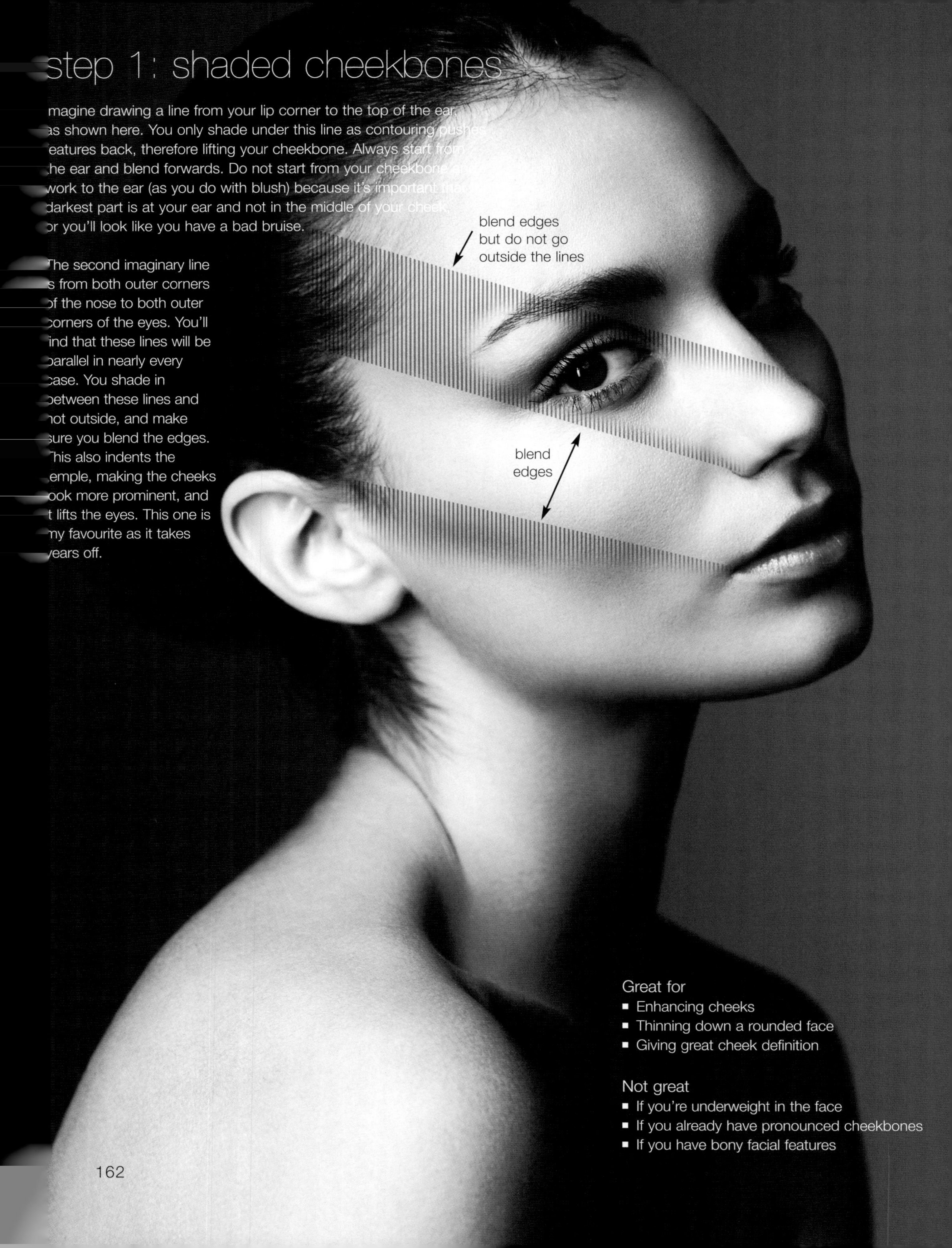

blend edges
but do not go
outside the lines

blend
edges

Great for
- Enhancing cheeks
- Thinning down a rounded face
- Giving great cheek definition

Not great
- If you're underweight in the face
- If you already have pronounced cheekbones
- If you have bony facial features

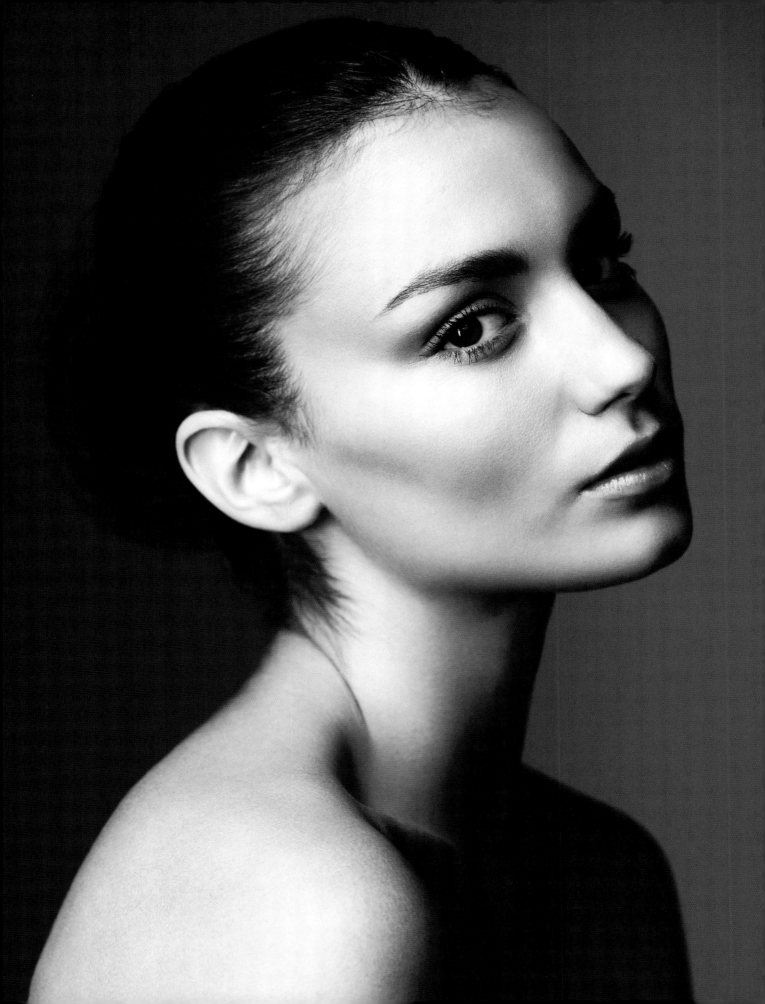

step 2: shaded hairline

This picture is self-explanatory. Just remember to blend colour into the hairline. I usually add more in the temple area. Make sure you blend the edges so they completely disappear. Don't use a product with any shine, and keep the shading in the middle of the forehead close to the hairline.

Follow the natural contour of your eye socket. You can go slightly above your natural socket if your eyes are ageing or if you have deep-set eyes. Using a matt brown shadow is great for this. Remember, this is not to create the look of wearing eye shadow (that's very '80s), it's to look undetectable. So keep it soft.

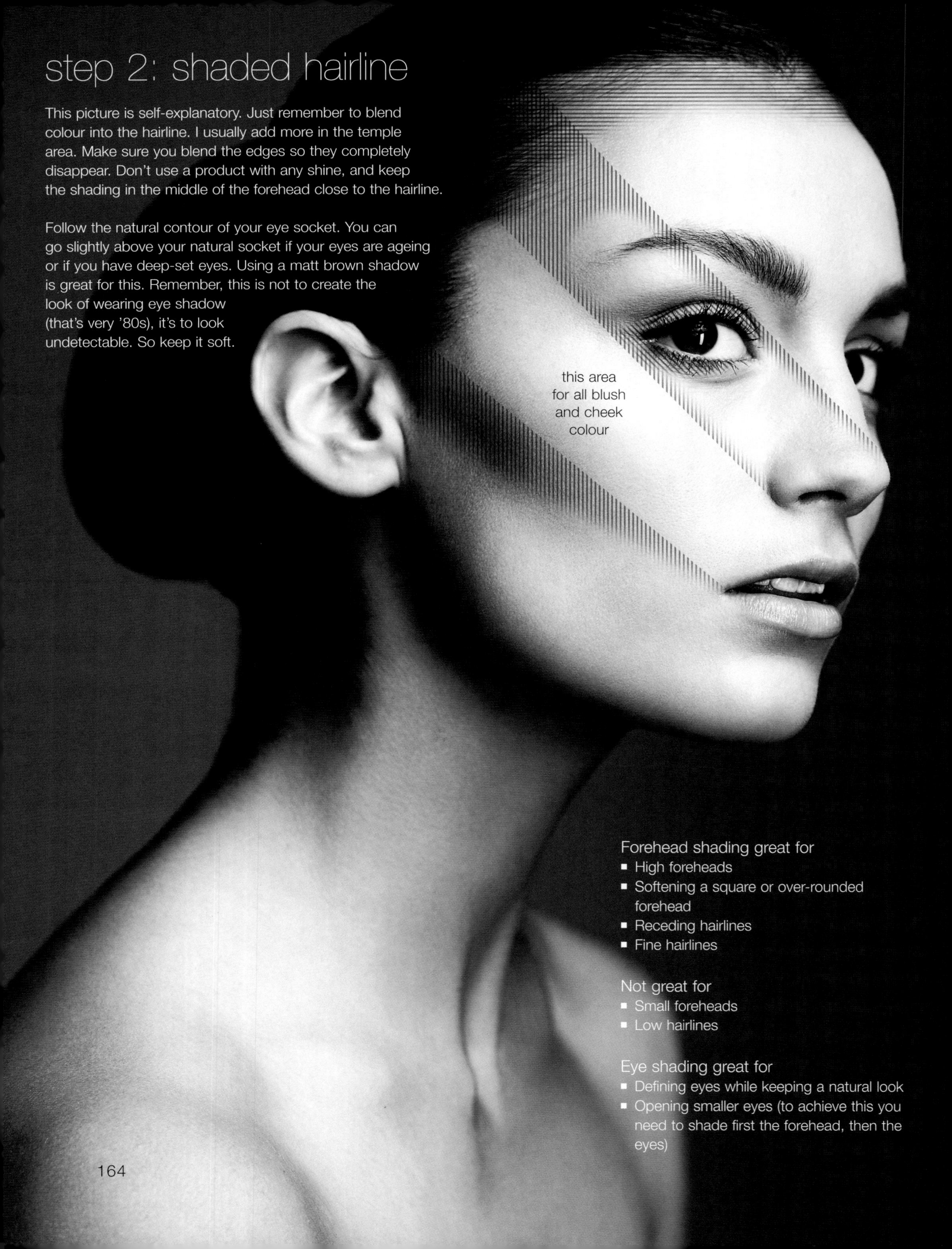

this area for all blush and cheek colour

Forehead shading great for
- High foreheads
- Softening a square or over-rounded forehead
- Receding hairlines
- Fine hairlines

Not great for
- Small foreheads
- Low hairlines

Eye shading great for
- Defining eyes while keeping a natural look
- Opening smaller eyes (to achieve this you need to shade first the forehead, then the eyes)

164

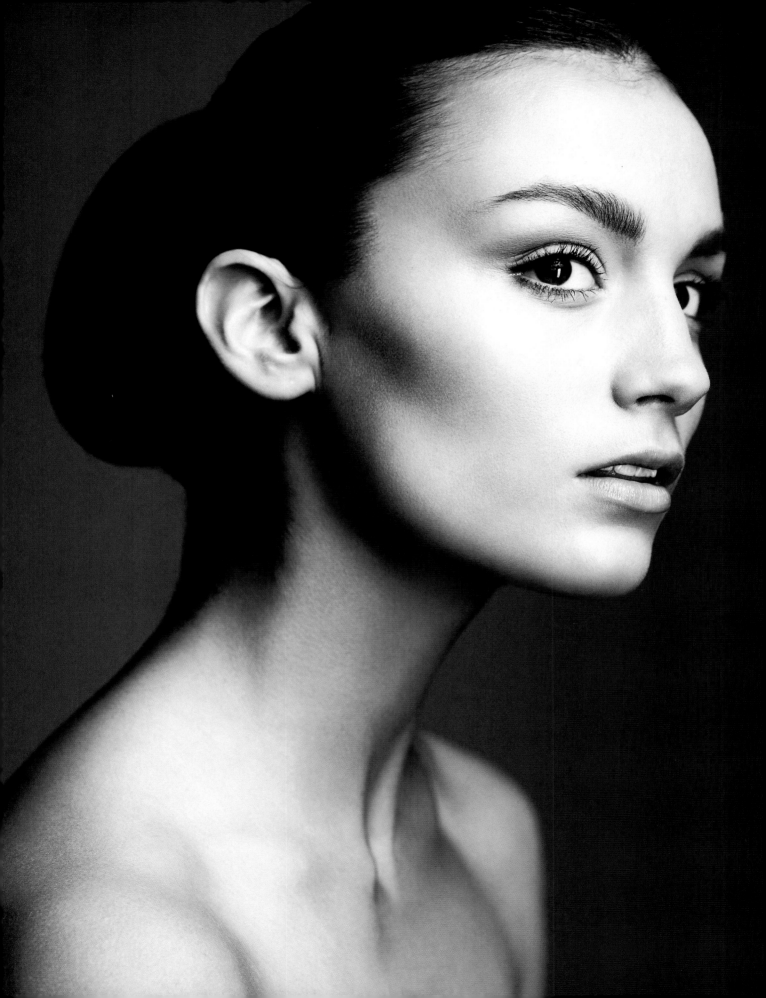

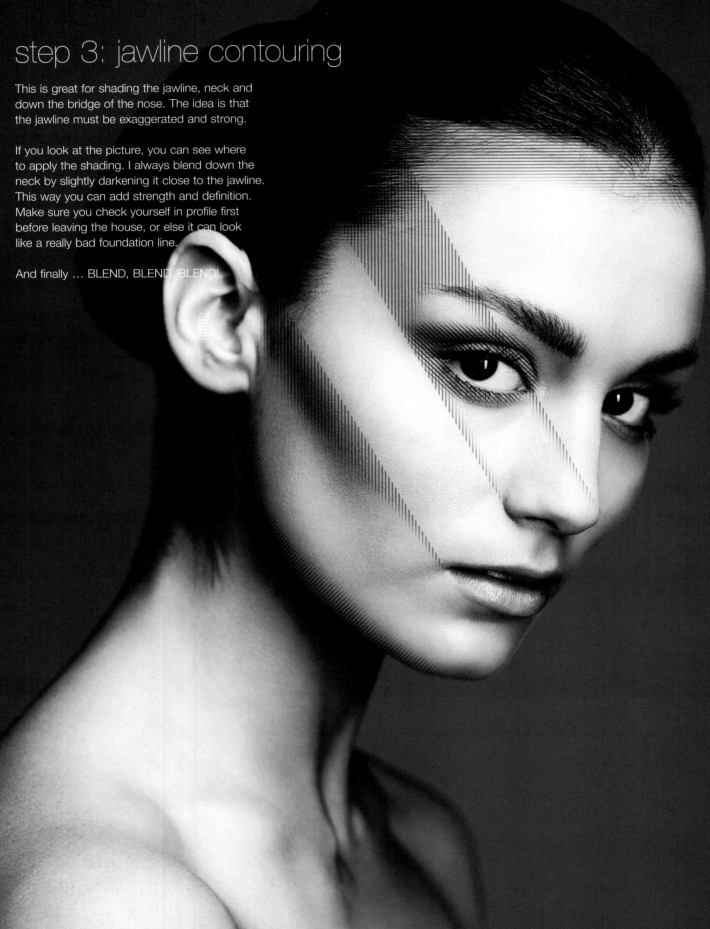

step 3: jawline contouring

This is great for shading the jawline, neck and down the bridge of the nose. The idea is that the jawline must be exaggerated and strong.

If you look at the picture, you can see where to apply the shading. I always blend down the neck by slightly darkening it close to the jawline. This way you can add strength and definition. Make sure you check yourself in profile first before leaving the house, or else it can look like a really bad foundation line.

And finally … BLEND, BLEND, BLEND!

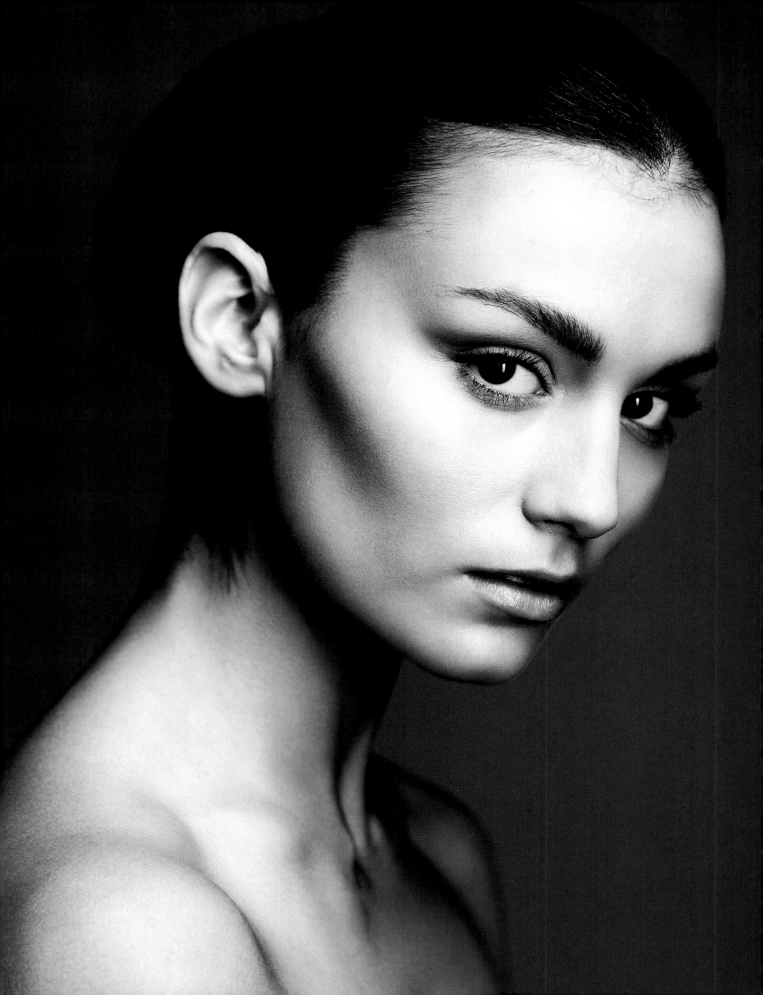

10 foundation

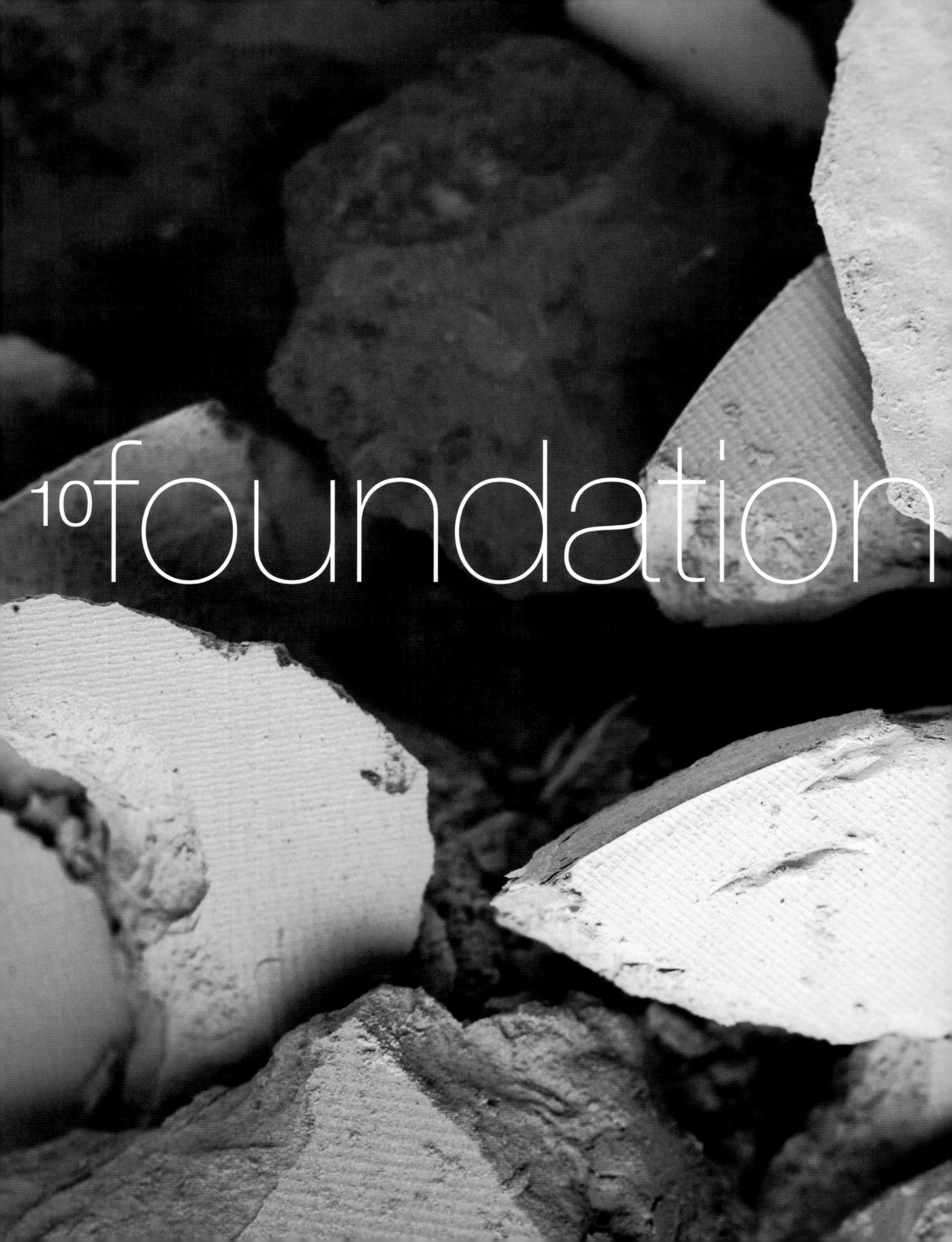

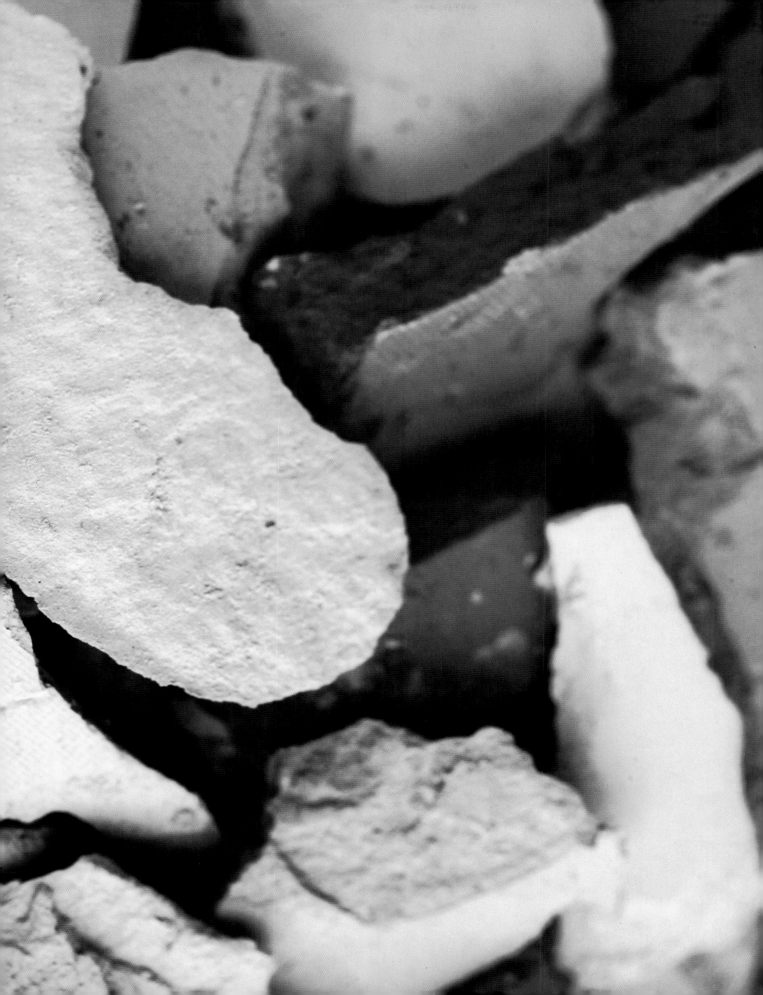

the facts about foundation

I find it hard to believe how many foundations there are on the market, not to mention what they promise and claim! Personally, I would like to see fewer 'claims' and more colour choices available … it's incredibly frustrating living in a multicultural country yet not being able to find foundations for dark or black skins, or anaemic pale shades (like myself). Some ranges carry them, but not many.

Also, it's so confusing when you find yourself at the department store faced with hundreds of brands offering everything from 'light-reflecting' to 'anti-ageing' to 'oil-controlling', and the list goes on. And to top it off, have you seen how many varieties of powders there are? Pressed, translucent, oil-free, sheer, silk, talc-free, etc.

So I'm going to simplify things for you. First of all, here is the list of what's available. Just skim through it and I will try to cut through the confusion.

Foundation types available

- **Liquid-based:** For all skin types (they can be either oil- or water-based—you must check).
- **Grease-based:** For dry or scarred skin, and mature skin.
- **Oil-based:** For dry skin or used for the effect of high-shine (I rarely use it—it just looks too greasy).
- **Water-based:** Great for sheer coverage and all skin types (perfect for hormonal, oily or blemished skin).

Textures

- **Matt:** It's very French (however, can look dated). Skin has no shine and powder is visible.
- **Velvety:** When the skin is semi-matt and the powder you use has a velvety sheen so it gives the skin a beautiful satin/velvet finish. This can be followed by the application of translucent powder.
- **High-shine:** This is achieved with an oil-based foundation used on skin that is heavily primed, allowing the skin's natural oils to come through. No powder is used. Sometimes vaseline or lanolin is used to accentuate the shine. This is a look used mainly for magazines and not an application I would suggest for a dinner out.
- **Luminous:** When shiny pigment or shimmery liquid has been added to the foundation to give it a pearlised, glimmering look. The skin can have a slightly metallic reflection (one of my favourites).

Types of coverage

- **Invisible (these foundations contain less than 50 per cent pigment):** Best used on really clear skin with not a blemish in sight. For invisible coverage use tinted moisturisers, water-based foundations with little pigment and some tinted sunscreens. With all these products you will achieve natural, flawless-looking skin.
- **Sheer:** Slightly more coverage than invisible. These foundations also give a natural look and suit skins with only slight pigmentation or subtle blemishes. This is the best foundation to have as it evens out the skin tone, and any other blemished areas can be attended to with concealer afterwards.
- **Medium:** Covers around 60 per cent of blemishes and uneven skin tone. In this category of foundation, there are many varieties to choose from, spanning luminous to matt and even oil to powder. I know this seems confusing. My advice is to go for water-based foundations with more pigment to achieve a dewy finish. When you want to cover the skin more, shy away from matt finishes in preference for a more luminous glow, which looks more like real skin as opposed to a mask.
- **High:** Sometimes you need this kind of coverage to conceal scars, birthmarks, severe acne, even tattoos. However, I would never use it as an all-over foundation as you can see it from a mile away and it doesn't look natural. I would most definitely opt for sheer-based foundation as an all-over cover then pull out your heavy-duty concealers when needed!

My golden rule when buying foundation

Never, ever match your foundation to your jawline, as your neck is the palest part of your body (the jaw blocks out sunlight to this area). Always match foundation to your chest area because your face and body must be the same colour. Also, when your body tans (either naturally or as a result of a fake tan), you must also darken your foundation to match. That is why I believe every woman should own two to three shades of foundation.

concealing blemishes

As mentioned before, this is not a book about skincare—there is a whole other book in that! And in any case, you can find most of the answers to your specific skincare needs on the net. But we all need to know what to do if we wake up on the morning of an eagerly anticipated social event with a massive blemish threatening to take over our entire face.

One of the things that aggravates blemishes is a moisturiser that contains oil (and most of them do). I have seen blemishes grow before my very eyes when a model arrives having applied an oil-based moisturiser, or any oil for that matter the night before. It's much like adding fuel to fire. If you have combination skin, ONLY APPLY MOISTURISER TO THE DRY AREA. There are so many products on the market today that are incredible at clearing blemishes. Some of the best are benzoyl peroxide, retinols, AHA, BHA and Stieva-A cream, which is my personal favourite—I use it all the time! (Also, new medications are now available for serious acne … so consult a dermatologist.)

Don't shy away from cosmetic doctors. They are my best friend—don't be scared! There are so many technologies being developed that will blow your mind, including Omni-Lux light therapy, lasers, micro-dermabrasion, ROLL-CIT, Plasma and many, many more. I have seen miracles! Patches of pigmentation removed within a week, and pimples and acne problems that disappeared completely. Capillaries and deep acne scars can be removed permanently. I only wish I had known about all this ten years ago—I would have saved a fortune, not to mention what it would have done for my self-esteem. The thing not to do is listen to the many myths that have been handed down for generations—most of which just don't work!

Things that don't work include

- Using toothpaste to dry out pimples. Fluoride can actually make pimples worse (straight from the mouth of a dermatologist).
- Breaking open vitamin E capsules, extracting the oil and applying it to the skin for healing. Vitamin E oil has been proven to cause dermatitis.
- Having facials where they use a lot of oil and massage—an absolute no-no for blemished skin.
- Using extreme drying products such as PURE alcohol. I have even been told that methylated spirits does the job—not true! You will only end up with huge burns that take weeks to heal.

Things that do work

One of my favourite remedies is drowning the blemish in whitening or red-reducing eye drops. Leave for as long as you can and rinse off before applying makeup. The only eye drops you can't use are ones that are tinted blue. I've learnt this the hard way—it takes away the redness all right, and leaves you with a whopping dark-blue bruise-type circle that will last at least a day.

After extracting a volcanic whitehead, apply hydrogen peroxide (7 to 10 per cent is the best strength) immediately. If you apply this twice on the first day the whitehead appears, it will sterilise the area to prevent further infection, reduce inflammation and stop the oil oozing out after extraction. Apply gently with a cotton bud for 10 seconds then wash off.

Step-by-step process to concealing blemishes
(in consultation with Dr Peter Dixon M.B. B.S. F.R.A.C.S.)

- **Step 1:** Cleanse the skin. My favourite trick is to mix bicarb of soda with a water-based cleanser (Cetaphil is my pick). This gives the most amazing exfoliation and is great for getting rid of the crusty dryness around the T-zone area, especially the nose. Treat it like you would a normal exfoliant and use only once a week. Just don't use this if you are already using an exfoliating product like retinol, Stieva-A, AHA or BHA and, particularly if you are on any acne medication.

- **Step 2:** Tone if you want. But, as a rule, I think toners are overrated and, guess what, contrary to what you might think, they can't close pores. Toners have a slightly different formula that rids the skin of excess oils, which is necessary for oily skin but rarely needed on drier skin. I use them when the skin has already been cleansed but is still oiled up and also on women who come to me after a long day at work en route to a social function, or on young girls on their way to a formal occasion when I don't have the time or the facilities to carry out the normal cleansing process. (You can also use alcohol-free baby wipes for these situations.)

- **Step 3:** The only product I use on a freshly cleansed skin is a water-based moisturiser or a makeup primer. Don't get sucked into applying rich lotions for this, that and the other before applying foundation because the foundation will just float on the skin and you want it to be absorbed into the skin. I have never known a top makeup artist to use more than one product before applying foundation. Trust me—I know! So when should you use a moisturiser? Always in dry skin conditions, but use a light, oil-free type.

To protect the skin in harsh conditions, use a moisturiser under a sunscreen but wash both off when you get home. You should also use one when travelling for long hours in airplanes, as they have a very dry atmosphere. The best time to moisturise is in the evening after you have cleansed the face and waited an hour if the skin is irritable. You can then apply a light moisturiser. The skin surface becomes damaged during the day and requires repairing, and it does this while we sleep. (Note: as the eyelids do not exfoliate naturally like the rest of the face, they have a thin skin and eye creams are nice to apply, but again, remember that the oils are only protective and not absorbed by the skin.)

- **Step 4:** After you have cleansed and moisturised, the next step is to apply foundation. You should not use concealer before you apply foundation because, one, it would be a waste of time as the act of applying foundation will remove the concealer, and also, you would end up using too much coverage as most foundations will actually cover 50 per cent of your blemish. Only after you've applied foundation should you apply the concealer to any areas which require it.

Types of foundation to use for concealing blemished skin

Only use two types of foundation. The first is water-based because it rarely causes any reactions and it gives a great finish. All skin types can use it (especially acne-prone skin) and it comes in different levels of coverage. And the second type is grease-based. YES, I said grease … not to be mistaken for oil-based.

Think of grease-based foundations as having the same texture as lipstick. It's not a pool of slime, it's more like wax. The reason I love it (and use it 80 per cent of the time) is that its formula is similar to the moisture that the skin produces, so it blends well and looks and feels just like normal skin. Also, the big catch is that as your foundation starts to wear off or as your skin gets blotchy or tired-looking, you can just massage it right back into place or, if needed, apply more. This is the one thing that is difficult with other foundations. For example, anything 'cream to powder' can be great in the short term, but if your skin is oily or you need to retouch your makeup, you really need to remove it completely and start again.

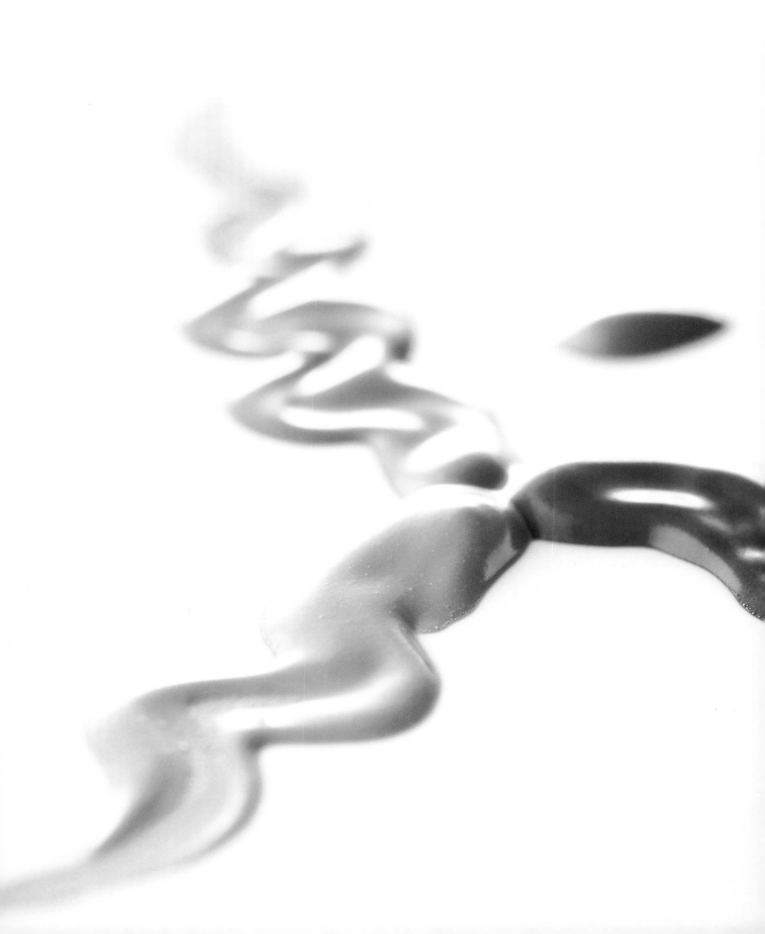

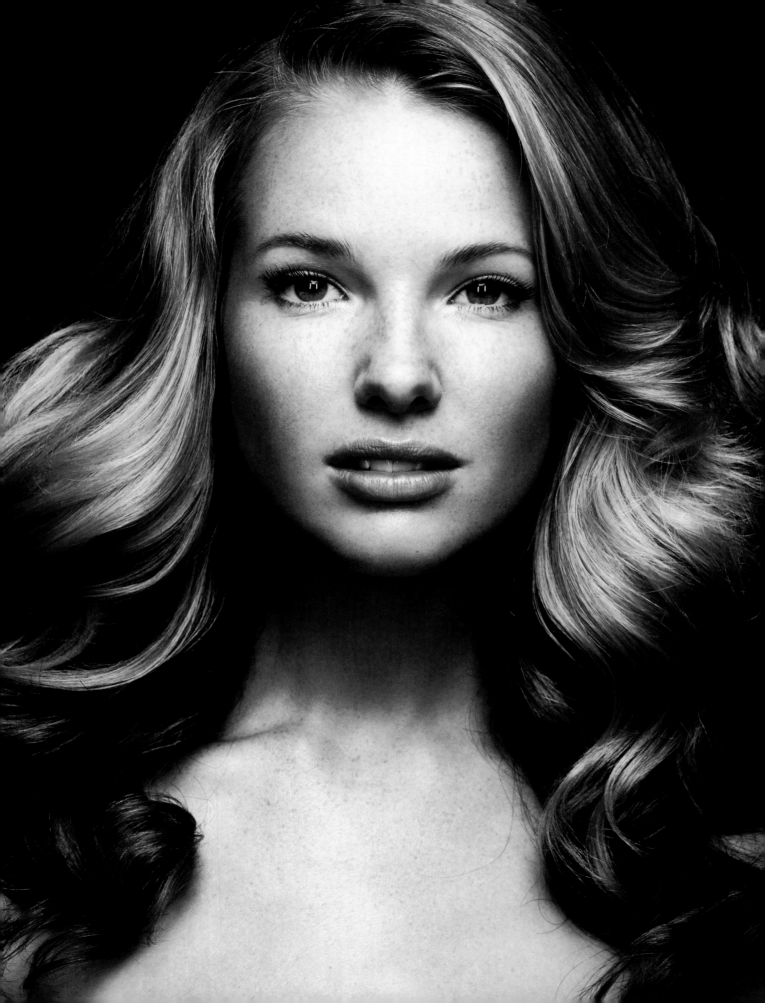

glowing

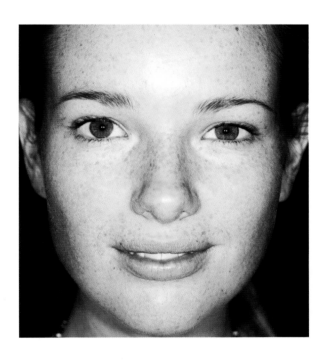

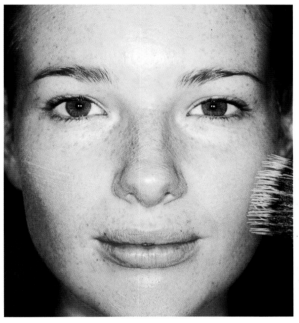

1 Prep the skin with bicarb of soda mixed with a water-based cleanser. This is the best (and the cheapest) exfoliant in the world, and it gives the skin an awesome glow. Then prep the eyes but don't powder.

2 Using a fibre-optic brush, apply a tinted moisturiser with sunscreen. Apply your foundation of choice, then lightly conceal any blemishes that remain visible.

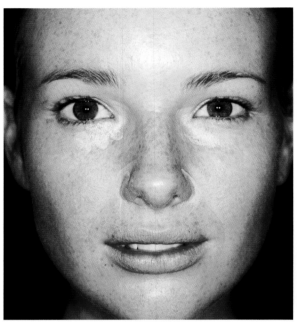

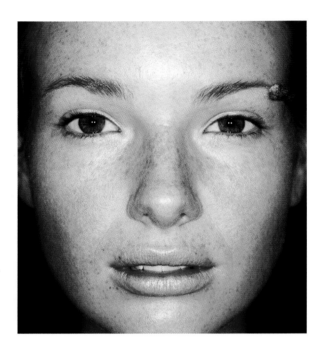

3 To give the illusion of wet, high-shine eyelids, apply a fine wash of a soft gold pigment to your lids using a wet brush. It's important to wet the brush to give the colour more intensity and stop it falling all over your cheeks. This is why powdering the eyes wasn't necessary when prepping — you want the pigment to stick. Be aware of creasing.

4 Using a highlighting shade that suits your skin tone, highlight the inner corner of the eye, under the brow, above the cupid's bow of the mouth, and in the centre of the bottom lip with a gold shimmer (see the Highlighting chapter on pages 196–202).

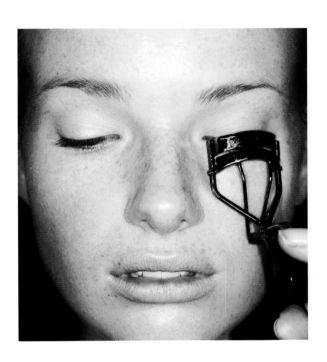 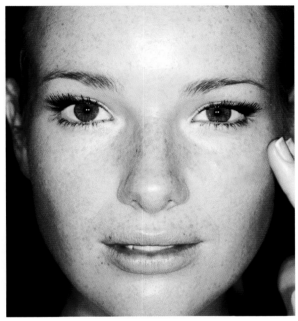

5 Curl the lashes. Apply a heavy set of single false lashes to the outside of the top lashes. You can see in this shot that Katie's skin is glowing.

6 Apply cream blush. I am applying it high on her cheeks and, importantly, Katie is not smiling. If you smile when you apply blush it creates wrinkles and you instantly age yourself. Then define brows and apply lip gloss. Finish off the look with some contouring of the cheekbones.

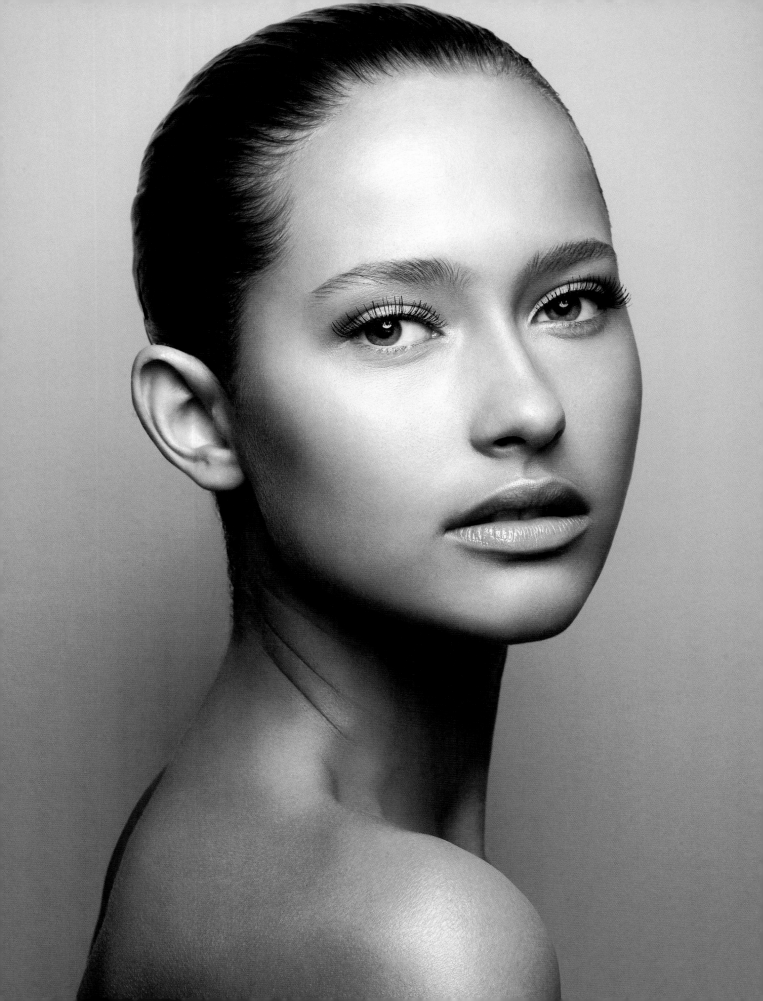

radiant

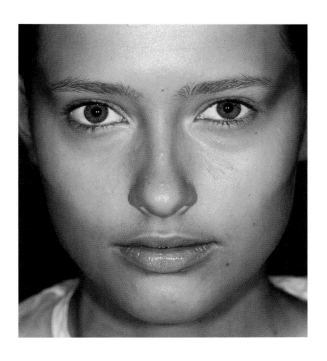 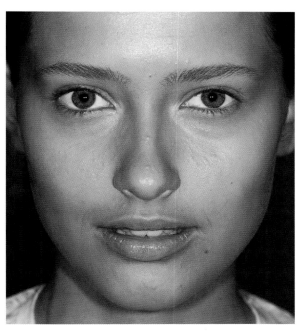

1 Mix an illuminiser with your foundation, and apply as normal. Then apply your contouring product and blend (see explanation in the Contouring chapter on pages 160–6).

2 Lightly apply corn-silk powder all over the face. Notice I have also applied lip balm on the lips.

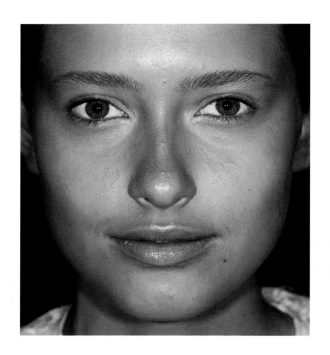

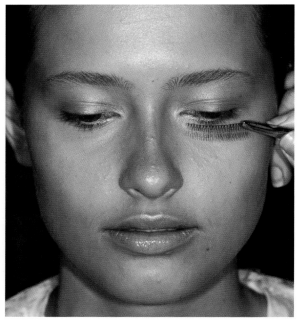

3 Highlight the face with a rose-gold pigment in all the highlight points, as explained in the Highlighting chapter (see pages 196–202).

4 Curl lashes, then apply nude false lashes to the top lashes. Once eyelash glue has dried, apply thick black mascara to the top and bottom lashes. Apply foundation over the lips, then a light gloss over the top. Finish by combing up the brows.

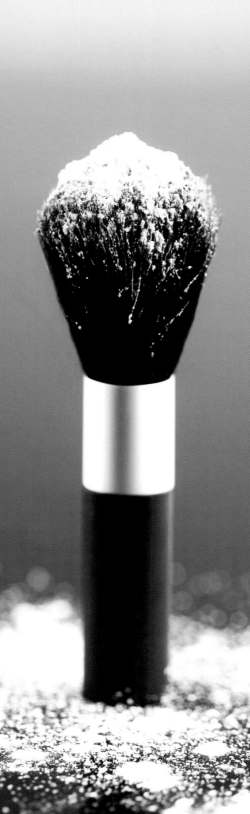

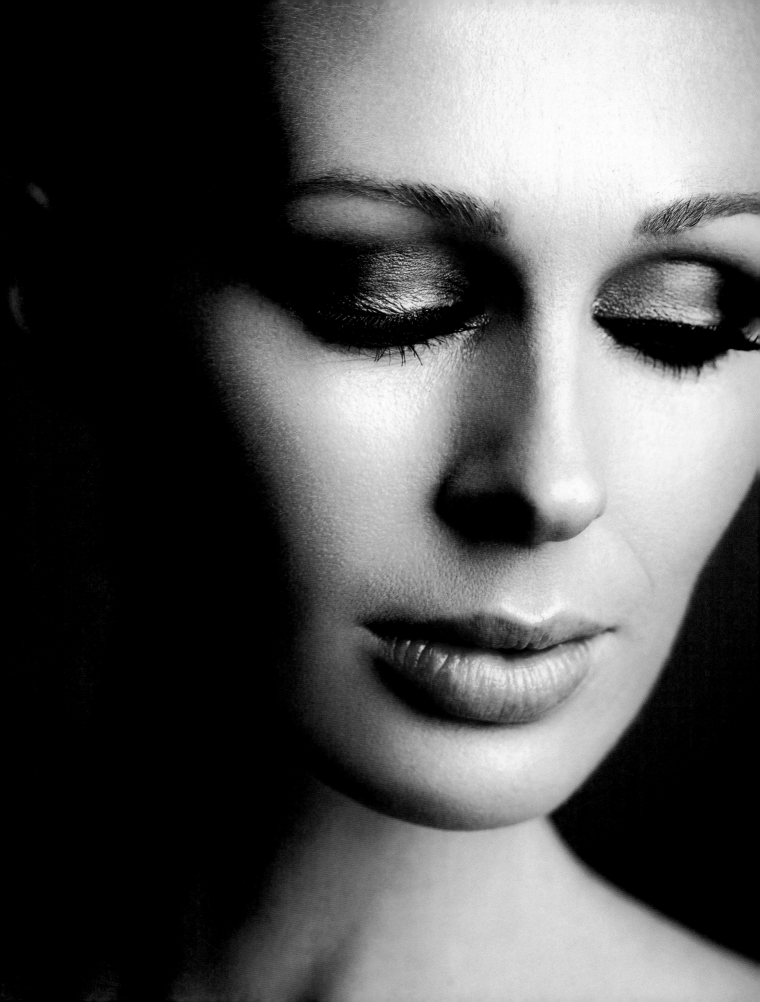

velvet

1 Match your foundation colour to your chest area. Using a brush, apply the foundation to your face, then blend with your hands. Treat the foundation as a moisturiser and as a first base.

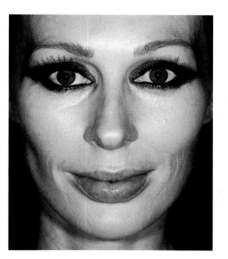

2 Lightly powder your face with sheer, translucent powder: remember, if you prep your skin correctly, the powder will look sheer and have a velvety finish. Lightly conceal blemishes if you need to. Define brows by filling them in with a light pencil and comb them up, then lightly powder for a velvety finish. If you want to use a bronzing powder you can now that you have powdered the skin, otherwise you must stick to a cream bronzer as it won't blend correctly, and will look uneven.

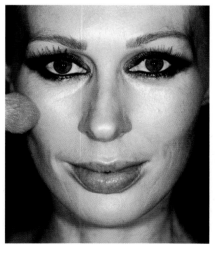

3 Finish by applying blush—I have applied a golden-pink blush. It is very important not to smile when applying blush. Notice I am applying it high on the cheekbones as it gives a more youthful look.

11 bronzing

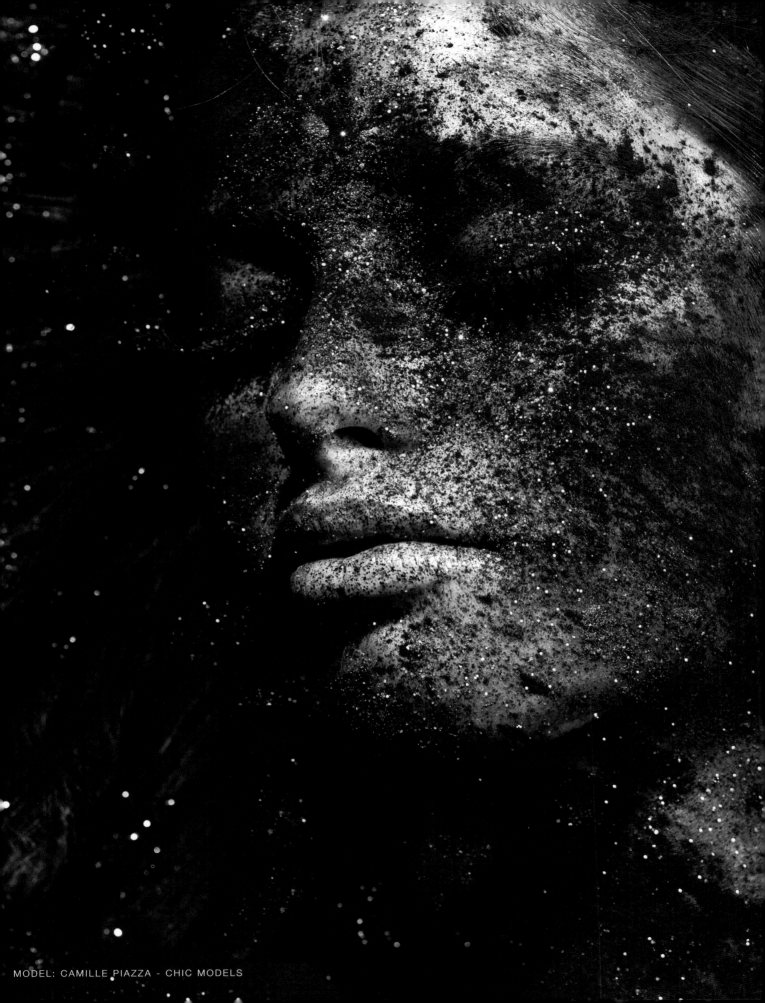

MODEL: CAMILLE PIAZZA - CHIC MODELS

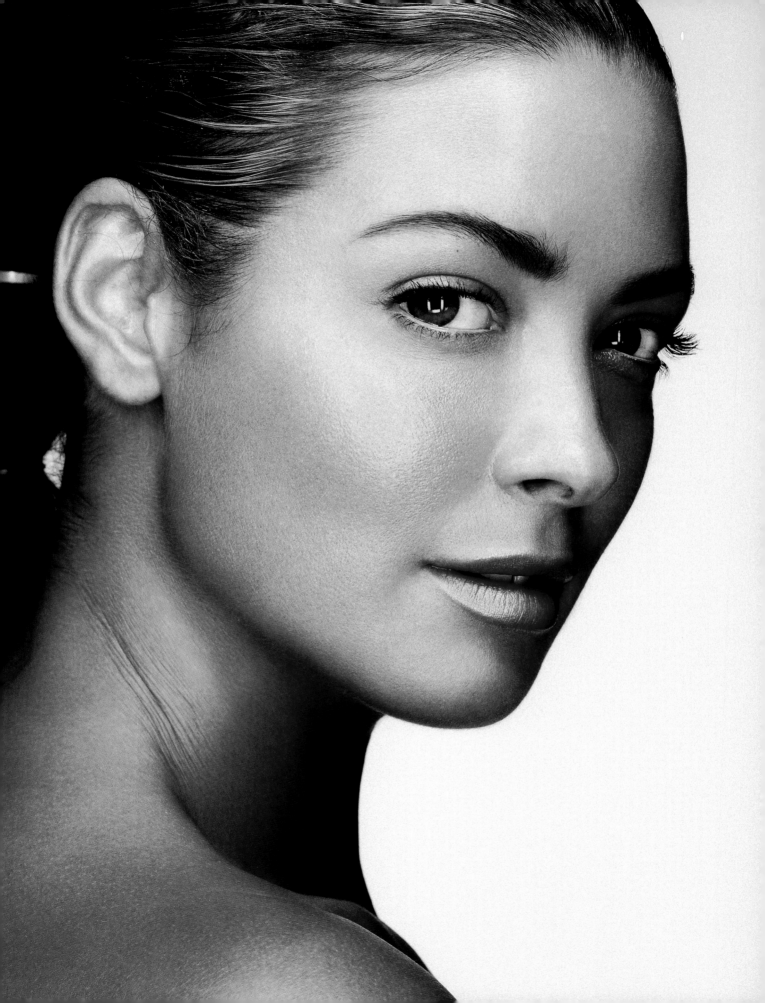

ooking suntanned means different things to different cultures. In the West, it means we can afford holidays, i.e. we have the time and money for overseas travel to an exotic island to soak up the sun. In the East, it means the opposite—working in the fields to provide for yourself and your family. In the past, this was frowned upon: if you had money in the East, you didn't need to work outdoors, you stayed in and had servants work for you. To this day, if you go to Asia you will find the cosmetic counters filled with whitening products.

Times are changing and most people now see tanned skin as something that ages you and gives you cancer, while the younger generations of Asian women are now embracing the healthy glow. So this brings us back to bronzing, that fabulous thing you can do yourself wherever you are, whatever time of the year.

Bronzing—yes, it's an obvious word, a very clear statement, meaning to bronze, to look like you have been on a holiday, to have a healthy glow. Not like you suffer from jaundice, drink way too much carrot juice or may have glandular fever. I rarely see women who get it right, basically because most of us don't really understand how the skin tans naturally. Skin never tans evenly. That's a fact. It's darker in some areas and paler in others. Most importantly, over the following pages, you should notice that as I make Jodi (our model) darker with bronzer, I darken her body colour to match.

This is the 'before' shot. If you look closely, you can see that Jodi's body colour naturally is one shade darker than her face. This is very common; we just don't carry the same amount of pigment in our face as we do on our body. That also goes for our hands, neck and feet (and stomachs, in some cases).

Using a fibre-optic brush, I have used a liquid foundation (sheer coverage) three shades darker than her face colour. Then I set it with translucent powder, and lightly contoured her cheeks and hairline (see the Contouring chapter on pages 162–4) with a matt bronze powder.

step 3

Using a kabuki brush, I have applied blush then added gold shimmer powder as an extra highlight to the top of her cheekbones (see the Highlighting chapter on pages 196–202). I have lifted the bronze high on her cheekbones and softly blended up her temples. I have used the same colour to apply a soft wash to her eye socket area. Just make sure the eyelids are well powdered beforehand for easier blending.

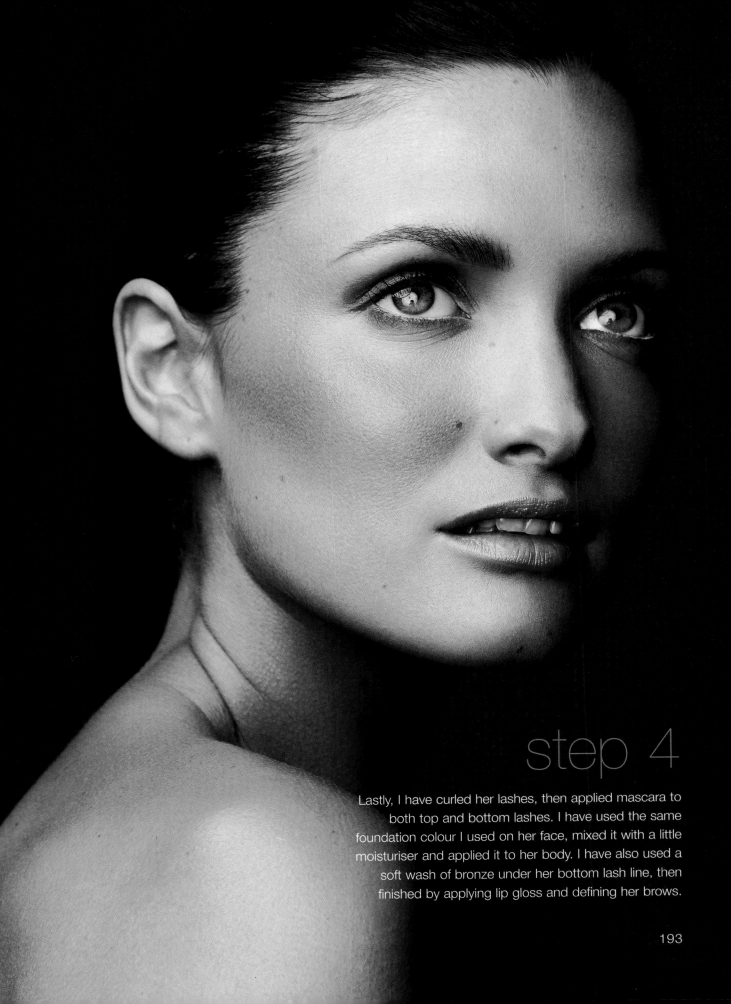

Lastly, I have curled her lashes, then applied mascara to both top and bottom lashes. I have used the same foundation colour I used on her face, mixed it with a little moisturiser and applied it to her body. I have also used a soft wash of bronze under her bottom lash line, then finished by applying lip gloss and defining her brows.

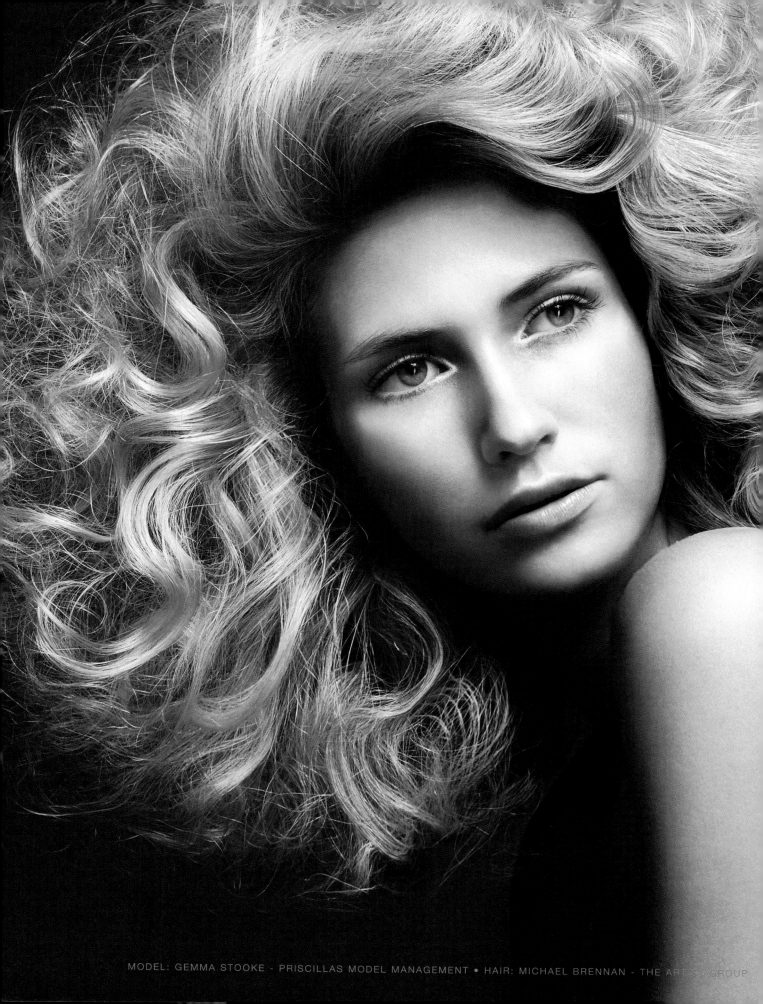

highlighting

highlighting is a technique that brings your face and makeup to life. It is one of the quickest ways to turn a basic makeup into a beautiful one. I don't know anyone on this planet who doesn't want beautiful, glowing skin. It looks sexy, expensive and very glamorous!

This technique works even for oily skin. Why? Because the skin has places where it should and shouldn't shine. Glowing up or highlighting the skin doesn't mean slapping on highlighter all over the face. This is a sure way to end up looking like a grease slick. When I talk about highlighting, I mean having special parts of your face that illuminate and glow, such as your cheekbones and the inner corners of your eyes.

To highlight successfully, you need to know:

- the right shade to use
- where to highlight
- where to never, ever highlight.

Never highlight:

- heavily blemished areas
- areas where you're conscious of lines and wrinkles such as the eyes and mouth
- on puffy eyelids
- excessively oil areas as they will shine anyway
- under the eyes.

What is the right shade?

The golden rule of highlighting is that the colour you choose must be the same as your skin tone or lighter, and must always have a shiny or shimmery finish.

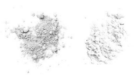

For pale skin:
off-white or any eggshell shade are best; gold will look too yellow on the skin (think Academy Awards statue—not attractive).

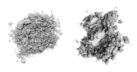

For medium-toned skin:
soft golds and rose golds are best—not bronze as it will throw too much orange.

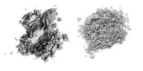

For dark skin:
golden bronze or straight bronze are best; never use pale, white or frosty shades.

For black skin:
burgundy bronze, dark shimmery chocolate or dark bronze.

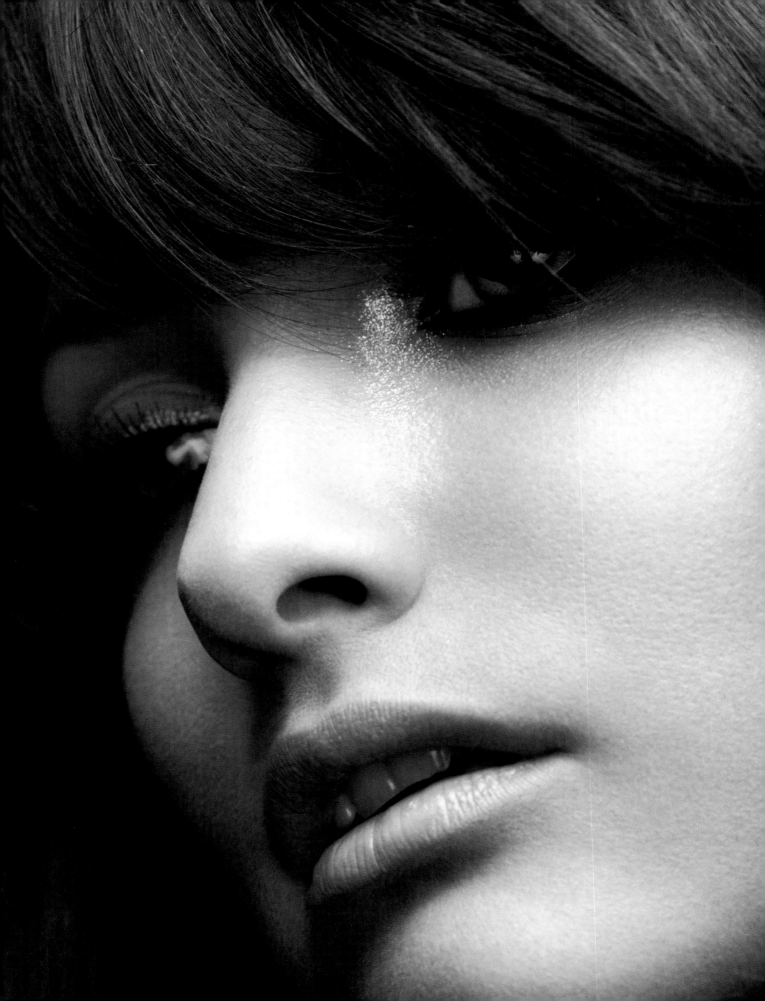

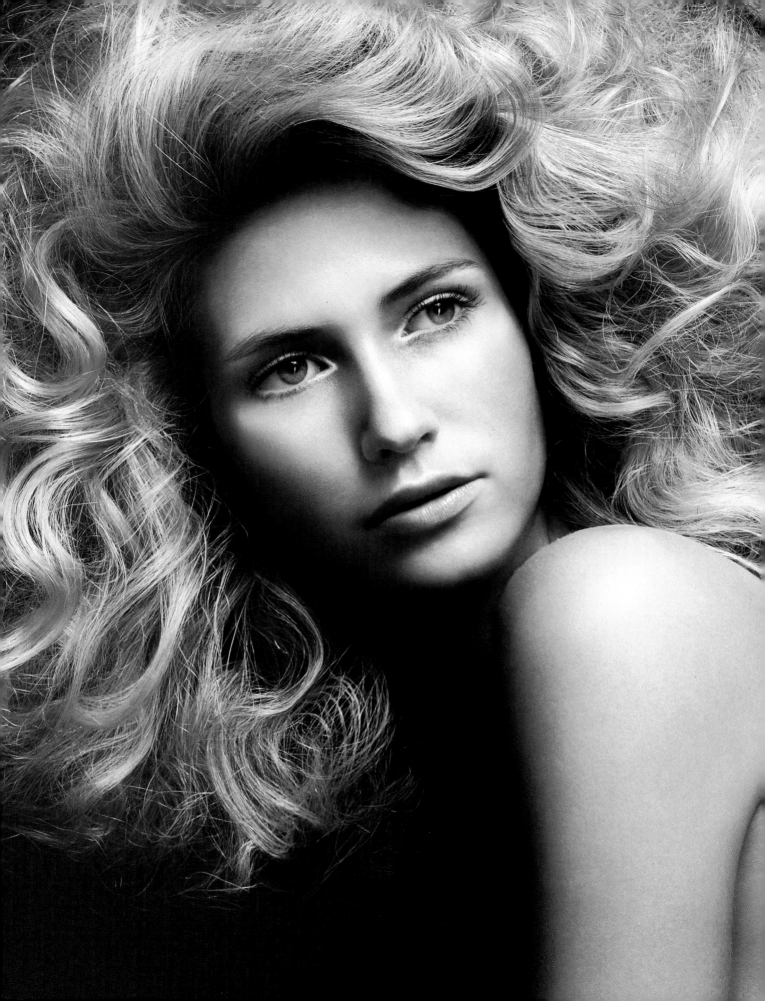

highlighting for pale skin

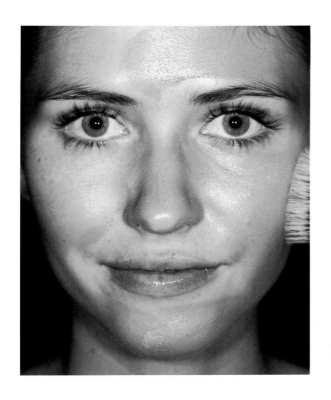

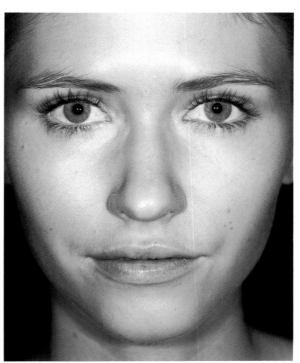

1 Mix foundation with illuminiser then apply to the face. I am applying the foundation two shades darker than Gemma's natural skin tone, matching it with her chest colour.

2 Conceal under the eyes after applying the foundation.

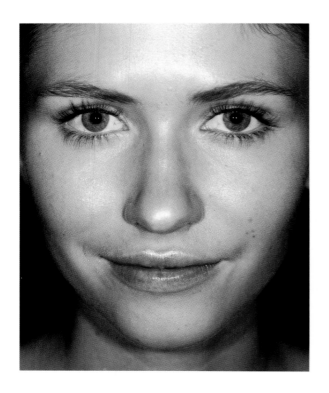 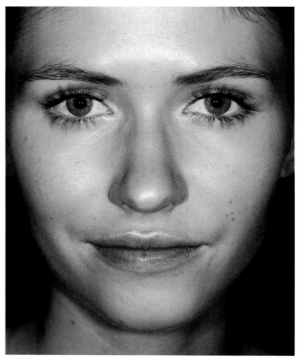

3 Highlight straight down the centre of the nose. If your nose is prominent, I wouldn't recommend this as it can make your nose appear wider. Apply gold eye shadow to the cupid's bow of the lip. This makes the lips appear fuller than applying lip liner.

4 Using a wet brush, apply gold pigment to the inner corners of the eyes, both top and bottom, one-third of the way along.

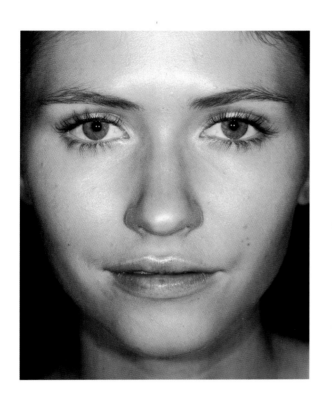

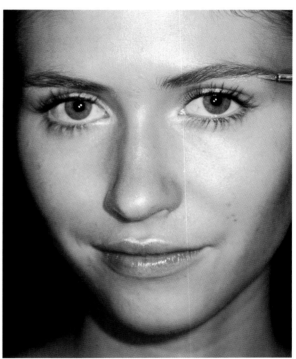

5 Apply the same wet gold pigment on the eyelids.

6 Also apply it underneath the eyebrows. Highlighting under the brows is beautiful because it catches the light as you turn from side to side.

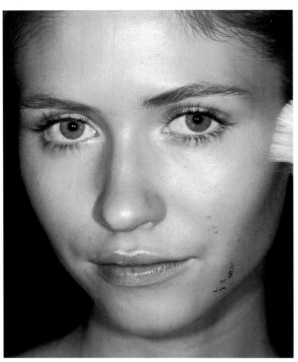

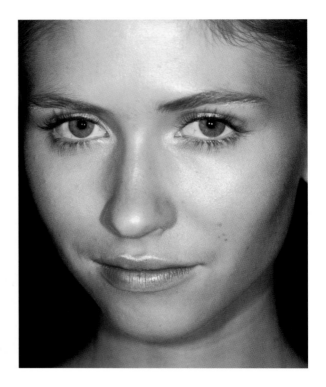

7 Using a feathery brush, apply a gold highlight to the cheekbones. This brush prevents the highlight on the cheeks from looking too heavy. Don't smile while applying it because smiling causes the cheek and eye areas to wrinkle, making a smooth blend impossible.

8 If your skin is dry, I would recommend applying shimmer powder on the centre of the forehead, and the chin. Just don't add too much as it can make the skin look oily.

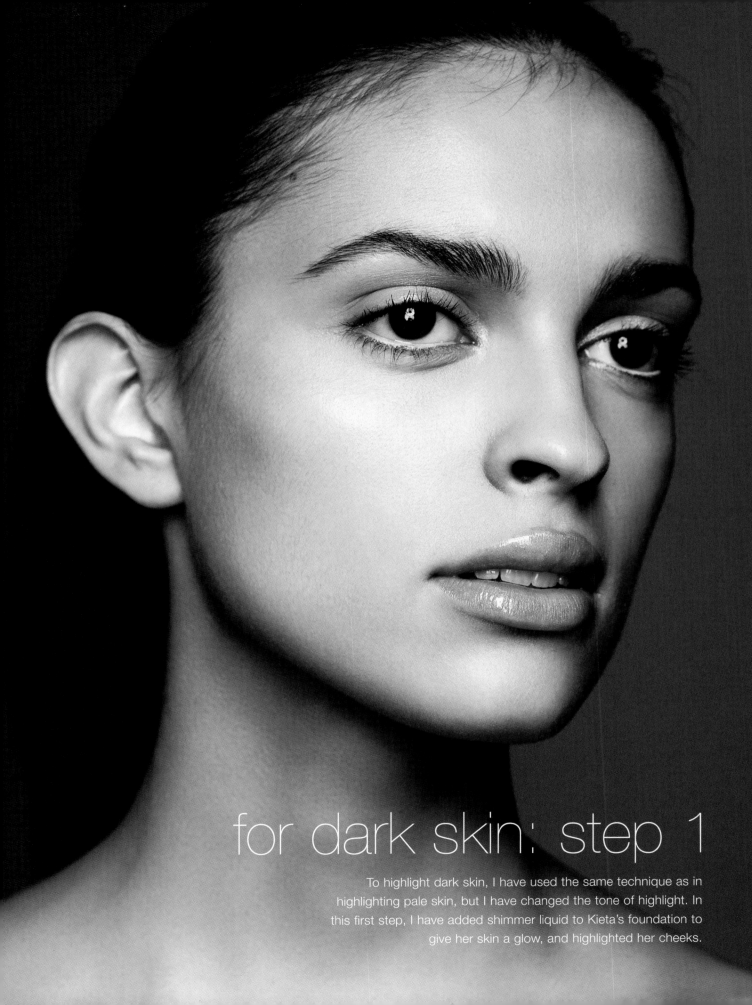

for dark skin: step 1

To highlight dark skin, I have used the same technique as in highlighting pale skin, but I have changed the tone of highlight. In this first step, I have added shimmer liquid to Kieta's foundation to give her skin a glow, and highlighted her cheeks.

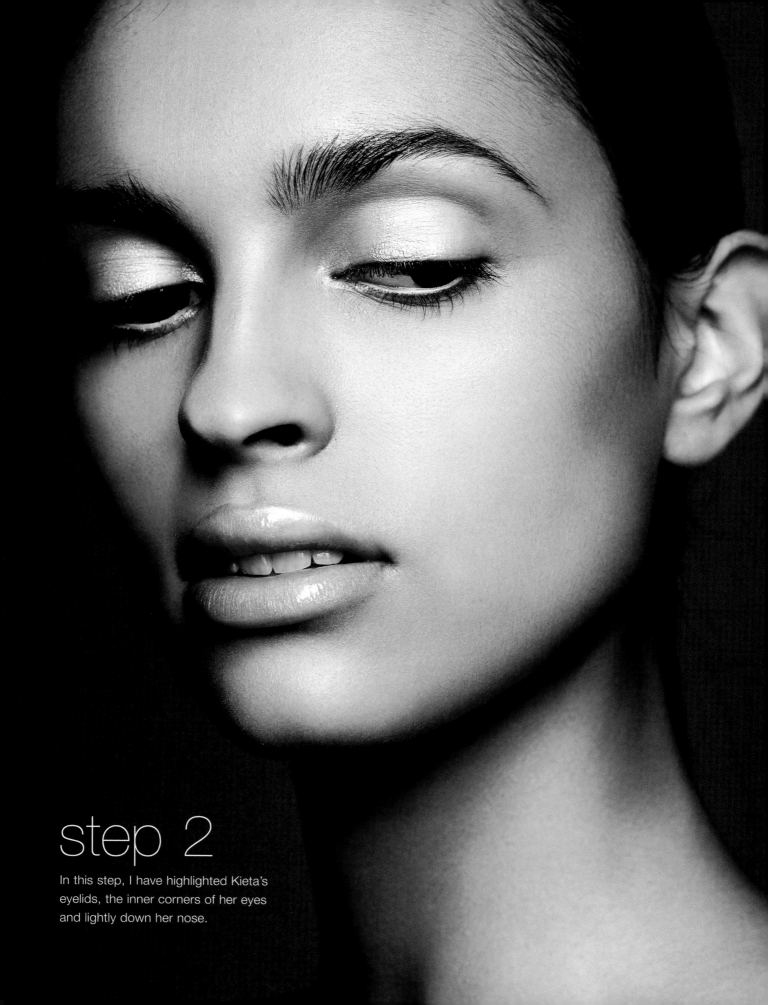

step 2

In this step, I have highlighted Kieta's eyelids, the inner corners of her eyes and lightly down her nose.

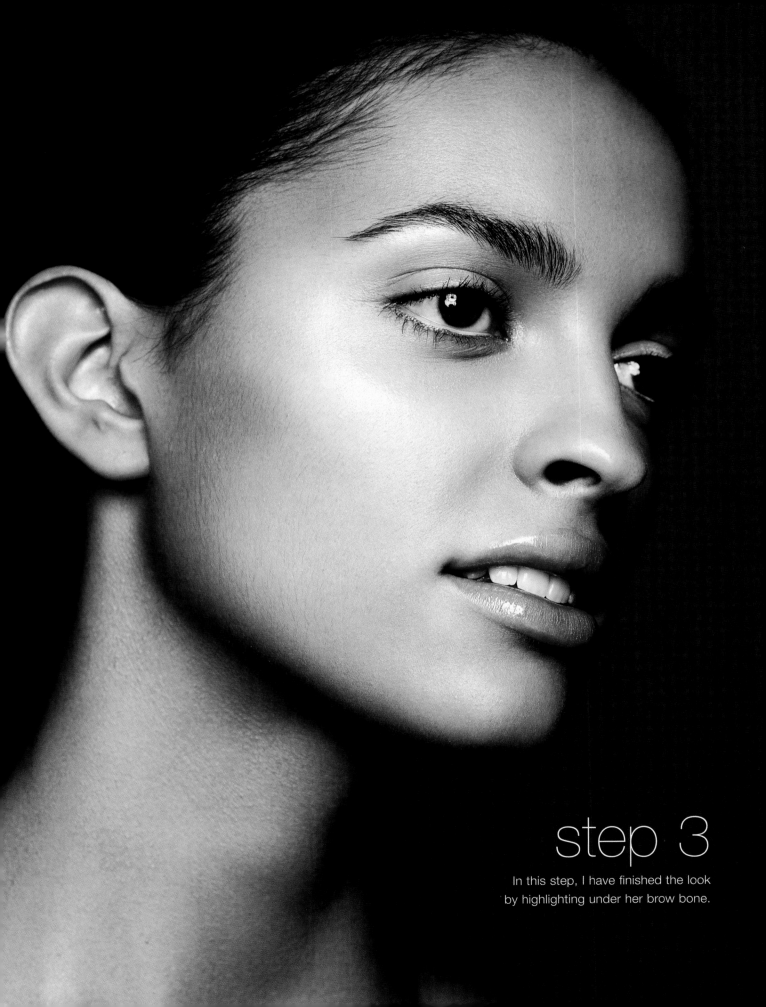

step 3

In this step, I have finished the look
by highlighting under her brow bone.

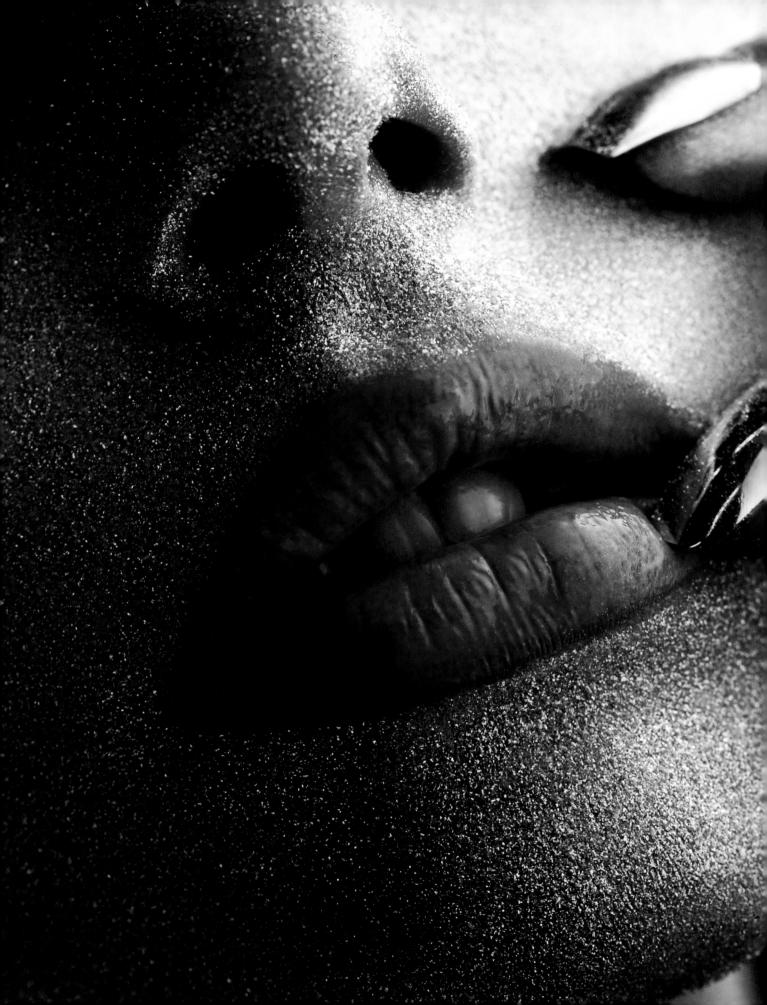

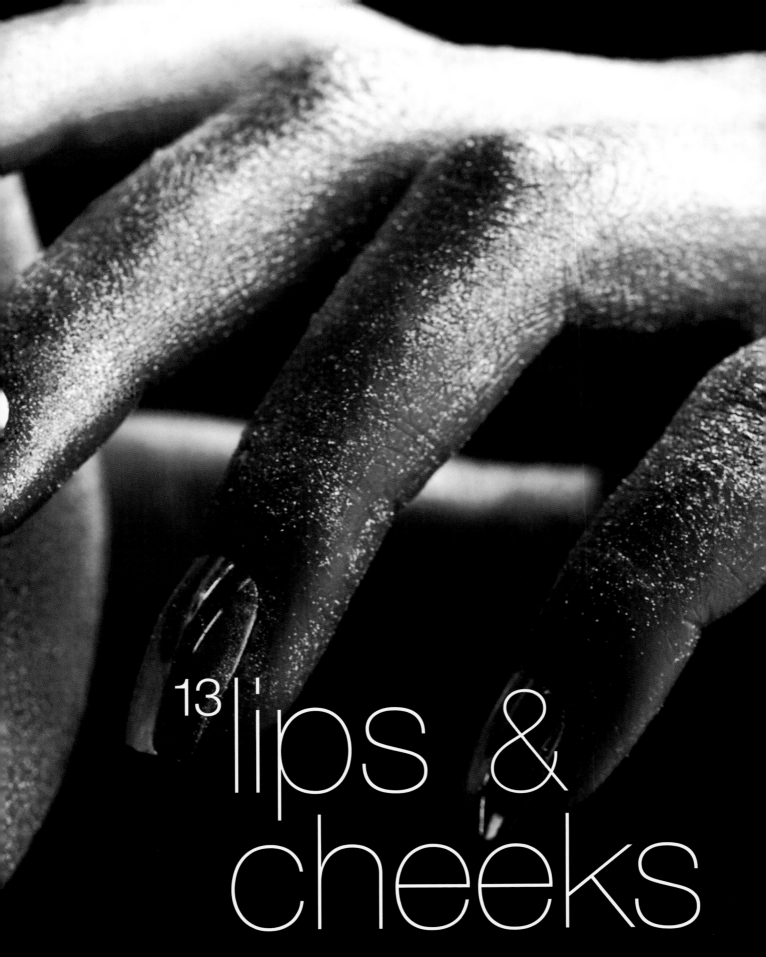

One thing I don't want to do with this chapter is teach women what they already know! Meaning, most women apply lipstick every day, and don't need to be told how to do it, and nearly every beauty magazine has some step-by-step or tips for making your lips bigger, smaller, glossier, etc. What I have done instead in this chapter is avoid all the norm, and show you some tricks of the trade: how we achieve some of the amazing lip shots you see in glossy magazines (I should know, I do most of them … I'm known to many as the 'lip queen').

Here are the questions I get asked the most

- Can my daughter do some work experience with you? (just kidding)
- What lip colour suits me?
- How do I stop lipstick from running or bleeding?
- What's the best way to make my lips look bigger?
- How do I choose quality lipstick?
- Should I use lip liner or not?
- What should I do about dry, cracked lips?
- Application: which is better? Brush vs. finger vs. lipstick tube?

Here are the golden rules

Finding the right lip shade

Here's the trick. If you have absolutely no idea, picture having two lipsticks sitting in front of you, and you have to choose one, like it or not! One is 'fuchsia pink', the other is 'tangerine orange'. Even if you detest both of them, you will find yourself detesting one less than the other. If you pick 'fuchsia pink', then in most cases you suit and wear 'cool' colours, as pink itself is cool.

So, if you pick the pink, you should always tend to look for cool or blue undertone shades, cool reds (verging on wine shades or even burgundy), all pink shades, pink-based nudes if you like the paler shades, and pink-based browns. And of course, absolutely nothing with orange or warm brown because these cool colours clash badly with warm tones.

If you picked the 'tangerine orange', the opposite is true. You would tend to wear gold jewellery if you're colour-coordinated, earthy clothing colours, creams instead of whites, burnt orange, caramels and even bright yellows. So if you pick the orange, you should go for all orange brick-based reds, anything warm in general, warm browns, peachy nudes, all bronze shades, and you can even pump up your lips with golds!

If you can wear both the pink and the orange (and actually get away with it!), you may fit into a very small category of women who can wear cool and warm. Lucky you! (Please, just not at the same time!)

If you are still confused and have no idea, then stick with anything in the wine shade, such as mahogany or plum. These colours are the only ones in the colour spectrum that are both cool and warm. This also goes for hair and wardrobe colours.

Another basic rule that you need to be aware of is that all cool-coloured lip shades, such as cool reds, all pinks and wine colours, will make your teeth look whiter, whereas all brown shades can make your teeth slightly yellow. Guess which is better?

Never use lip liner that's a completely different colour to your lipstick

If you want to use lip liner (I rarely do because I can get a perfect lip line using a brush if I want to create a sharp, precise edge), make sure you pencil in the whole lip. This is just for when your lipstick fades, so you're not left with an '80s lip line.

If your lips are naturally lined (or wrinkled), don't overuse lip gloss

If you do this, your lips won't just bleed, they will haemorrhage! Go for velvety or more matt-textured lipsticks instead. You can always apply a little gloss to the very centre of your lips only.

Never use too much lip gloss

Otherwise you will look like you're drooling; particularly in side light.

If you have lip hair, REMOVE IT

Don't bleach it. Even if the hair is blonde, it still grows down into the lip line, making it impossible to create a sharp edge. Many is the time that I have had to pull out the tweezers on models and rip out the hair so that I can perfect their lip line.

In my opinion, hair-removing machines are the best, because unlike wax they don't remove any skin. I don't like hair-removal creams because of what they do to the skin. You can't take a product that removes and dissolves 'hard keratin' (such as hair) without affecting the more sensitive 'soft keratin' (skin) beneath.

Don't apply foundation on your lips or under lipstick

Yes, we do sometimes use foundation as lipstick to create a nude effect. But putting it under a lipstick can get you into trouble. You end up with a white cakey line all around your lips because foundation and lipstick can be made of opposite components (e.g. water vs. grease), so they won't blend together. Not a great look, believe me. If you want nude-looking lips, buy a nude lipstick.

Dry lips: how to exfoliate

I like to load up the lips with pure, clear lanolin. This is also sold as 'nipple cream', by the way. Don't use white lanolin, though, as it's been mixed with water and gives you that I'm-wearing-zinc-and-taking-up-cricket look.

If you let your lips soak in moisturiser first, it allows the dead skin to soften, making it easier to remove it. Then mix bicarb of soda with a water-based cleanser and scrub away gently. Next, reapply the lanolin, let it soak, then apply your lip colour.

If you're using a matt shade, don't moisturise beforehand. You can always apply a little afterwards if your lips are too dry.

How to choose the right lipstick for you: the trick cosmetic companies don't tell you

Have you ever tested a lipstick on the back of your hand, and loved it, only to get home and realise that on your lips it's a completely different colour? Or do you use up half the lipstick rubbing it back and forth on your hand until finally it's the colour you like? You guessed it: when you take it home you're also going to use up half of it, rubbing it back and forth until it's an inch thick and you can reach your desired tone. Well, let me make it simple. Use your fingertip if you can't test directly on your lips. Yes, your fingertip. Why? Well, have a look at the difference between your lip colour and the back of your hand. They are completely different. Your lips have a blue/red tone, and most people have a colour on the back of their hands that replicates a nude/neutral tone. So try a soft red tone on the back of your hand and look at how intensely bright it looks, then try it on your lips and you'll notice that it's very different. Your fingertip is a similar (well, a lot closer) texture and colour to your lips. So the colour you see on your fingertips is the colour you'll achieve on your lips.

How to choose the right nude

I love this question, because I see so many women getting this one completely wrong. Is it a nude lip you're aiming for, or is rigor mortis setting in? Pasty nude lips are a technique we teach in special effects makeup. To make someone look cold, ill or dead, we just lighten the lip paler than the skin tone and make it a cool shade. And *voila*, you're looking pretty dead!

Some women need lip colour, some don't. So how do you know? It's simple—without a scrap of makeup on, pull your hair back from your face. Now nude down your lips with foundation. If you start to look ill, don't go there. It is only possible to wear this look if you have full-on smoky eyes or other dramatic eye makeup. If you nude out your lips and your eyes come alive, be happy. You can successfully wear a nude lip and look sexier than ever.

But there are some rules:

- No dry lips allowed. If you have dry skin on your lips, exfoliate (see above).
- Never choose a lip colour paler than your skin tone. It should always be one to two shades darker.
- Remember if you're cool or warm (cool nudes can appear paler than they look and will be disastrous for anyone with a warm skin tone).
- Yes, you can use foundation to achieve nude lips, but your lips have to be nice and moist and so use only grease-based foundation.

Some great tips for lips

- If you want to make lipstick last longer, use lip gloss more in winter (because of the drying effects of the weather), and sticks and stains in summer.
- In most cases, when we do our makeup we save our lips till last. So a good tip is to load up your lips with lanolin or your favourite lip balm and then leave them while you do the rest of your makeup. This softens them, and by the time you've done the rest of your makeup, they'll be moist and luscious.
- Put your lip pencils in the freezer before you sharpen them (yes I know, an oldie but a goodie).
- Test lipsticks on your fingertip to get the true colour before you buy them. It's much closer to your lip colour and the skin texture is very similar.
- To create a fuller lip, first apply a highlight colour to the cupid's bow then apply your lipstick. This is quite simply the best trick in the book!
- You can also make your bottom lip look fuller by lightly shading just under your lip with a shading colour.
- Powder lightly around your mouth first (not on the lips) if you have a tendency for lip bleeds.
- Carry wipes with you if you're going out. If your lipstick looks old, dry, or as though it is an inch think, don't be lazy and reapply. REMOVE IT and start again.
- You cannot get a straight line around your mouth once the tube of your lipstick has lost its sharpness. You must use a brush.

How to achieve full lips

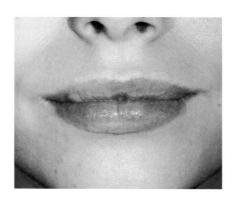

1 Lightly exfoliate your lips and apply lip balm. Apply foundation then lightly powder around the lip line (not on the lips).

TIP

With these steps, I'm going to show you how to achieve bigger lips without using a lip liner. In my whole makeup career, I've used lip liner maybe once.

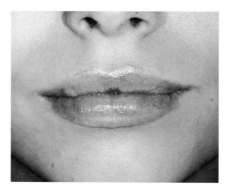

2 Using a shimmer powder, highlight the top of the lips, also known as the cupid's bow (see the Highlighting chapter, page 200). This instantly gives you a fuller top lip and defines it.

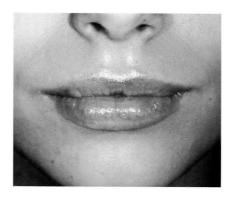

3 Highlight the two natural lines under your nose that join the cupid's bow. Some women love this technique, and some don't. As you can see, this area is more prominent instantly after application.

4 Using the same highlighter pigment, highlight the middle of the bottom lip. This creates roundness and a fuller bottom lip. I always do this after I apply lipstick. However, if you want a sexy nude lip, just use this technique then apply sheer, clear lip gloss. See how much fuller the lips are now—and we haven't even picked up a lipstick yet.

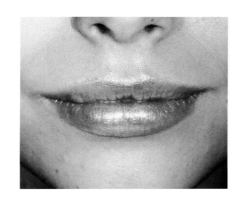

5 Now, you can stop here and leave your lips as is for a more matt finish, or you can apply clear gloss (but don't apply the gloss if you follow the next step). And my brush is larger than normal; I use the side of the brush to create my sharp line.

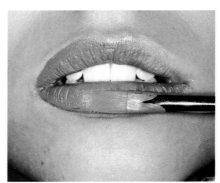

6 I have reapplied a shimmer powder to the middle of the bottom lip. See how much fuller and flattering the lips look? You can also use gold lip gloss to achieve this effect, then apply clear lip gloss. Note: don't apply too much to the outer edges, as you can look like you're drooling if the side light catches you.

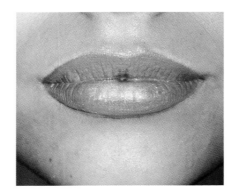

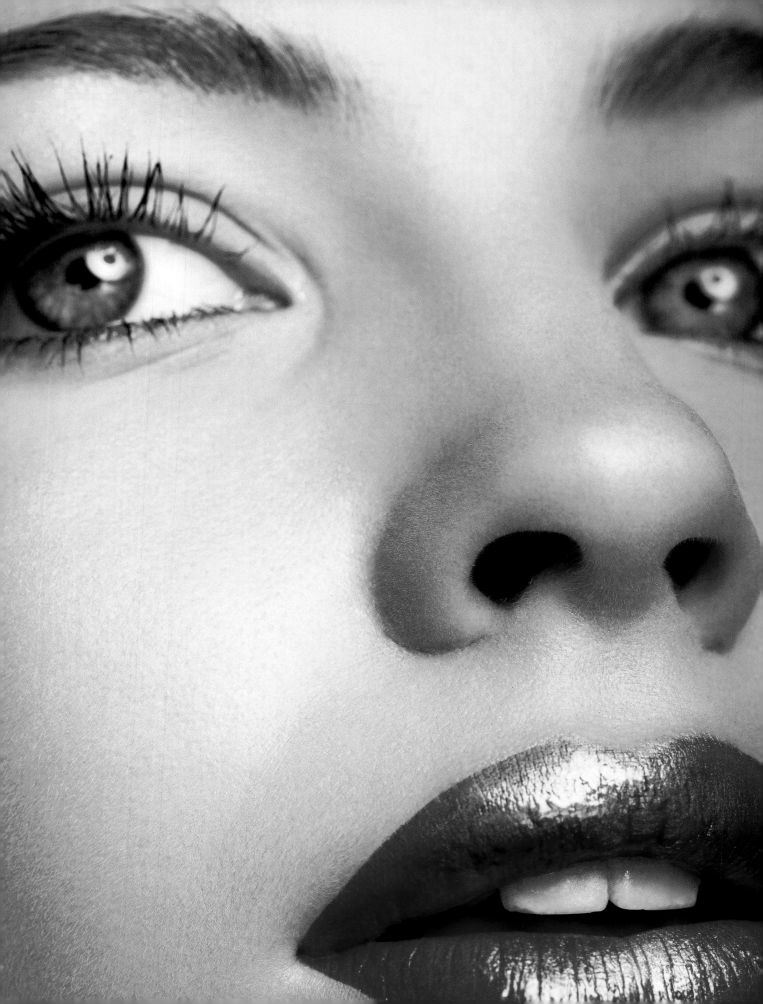

luscious lips

1 Prep the lips by exfoliating and moistening. To ensure lips are extra smooth, use bicarb of soda to exfoliate. Then apply a lip balm and remove after 5 minutes. Lips cannot be too wet for this to work. Apply a gold pigment to the cupid's bow of the lip.

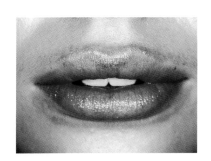

2 Using a bright fuchsia pigment on a brush, apply to lips. Because we are using an eye shadow, don't lick your lips or have them too moist before applying. You want the lips to have a similar texture to your eyelids so the pigment grips.

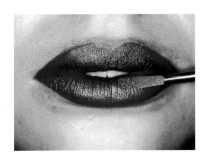

3 Apply a purple pigment to the top inner lip, and lightly to the bottom lip.

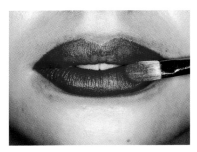

4 Finish by applying a gold pigment to the lower lip.

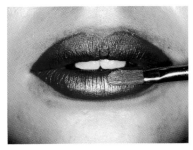

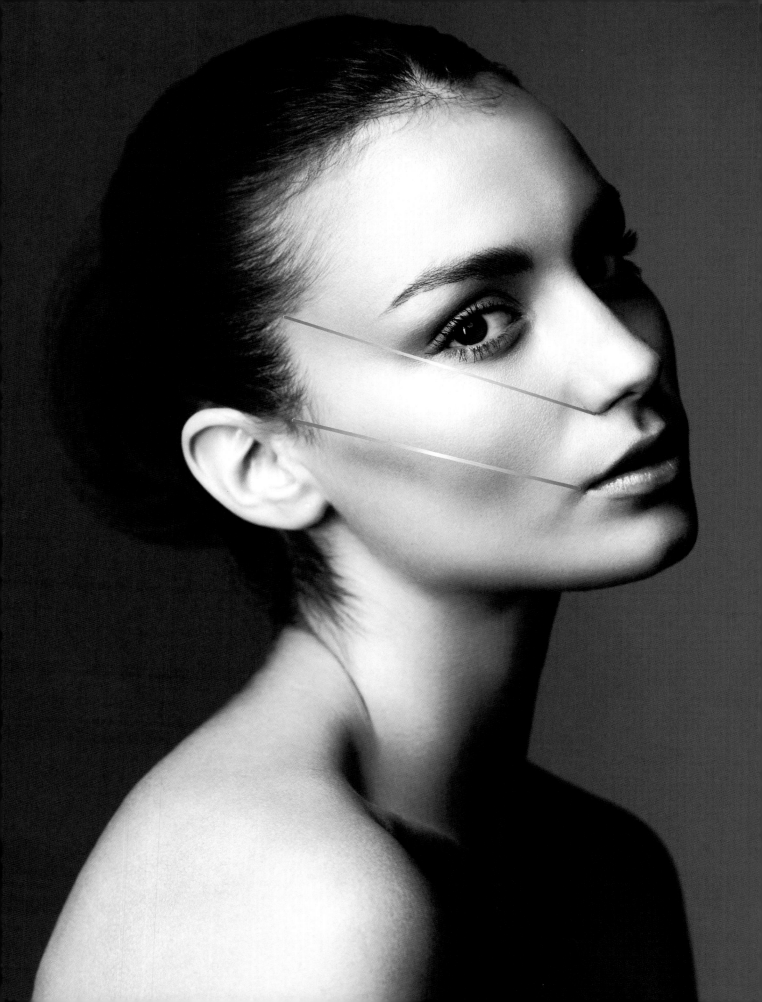

cheeks

Blush is the best product to bring youth and glow to the skin. However, if used incorrectly, it is also the best product to make you look like a clown ready for a fancy dress party. In the blush family, we have creams, powders and stains, and all are suitable so it's really a matter of personal preference. In the shot opposite (which you will recognise from the Contouring chapter), I have clearly outlined the area where blush is to be applied.

My advice is to always use a cheek colour that has some sort of sheen or highlight because cheeks need to have a glow. Even if you hate shiny skin and powder yourself to death, matt cheeks are so unattractive because matt blush flattens the cheek area and it ages you. The only time a matt blush comes out of my kit is if someone has oversized cheeks, and I want to to minimise this area.

The simple rule (and it's the same for eye shadow) is that you can only use cream blush on a creamy skin (i.e. skin that has had a dewy, liquid or cream-based foundation applied to it) that hasn't been powdered. And you can use powdered blush only on powdered skin. Remember, if you are using a powdered blush or bronzer, but hate face powder, just translucent-powder your cheeks first for blending purposes.

Brush size is important. The smaller your cheek area, the smaller your brush needs to be. The kabuki brush is the best for this area.

The golden rule is:

NEVER, EVER SMILE WHEN YOU APPLY CHEEK COLOUR. It ages you instantly, and yet every woman I know does it. The reason for this is that when you smile, you create tiny lines around your eyes, which the cheek colour cannot penetrate. So, when you relax your face, you are left with lines that look like wrinkles. Also, when most women smile, the muscle that protrudes is not necessarily your cheek muscle, so if you apply colour to this area when smiling, you'll notice that when you relax, that area will fall back closer to your mouth than your cheekbone. Cheek colour needs to be high and closer to your eyes than your mouth. Think of how teenagers get that sun-kissed glow—it's always really high up on the cheekbones, not halfway down the face near the mouth. In fact, placing cheek colour low on the face, is a technique used for ageing.

how to apply blush

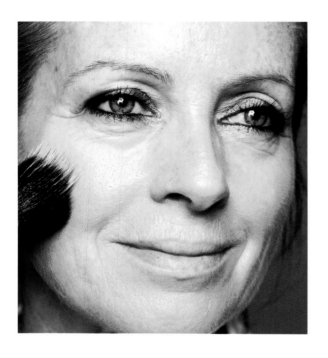

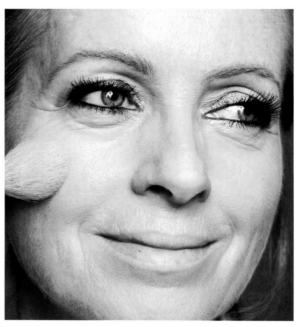

1 I have matched Sarah's foundation colour to her chest colour. You can see I am making the application with a round fibre-optic foundation brush. I have used a liquid foundation that has a slight sheen to keep her skin looking luminous, fresh and young.

2 Using a kabuki brush, I am applying corn-silk powder (it's the finest powder on the market) to create a velvety texture on the skin (fine translucent powder is your next choice). If you don't have a kabuki brush, my second choice would be a cotton pad because standard powder brushes are too spikey and leave imperfections on the skin.

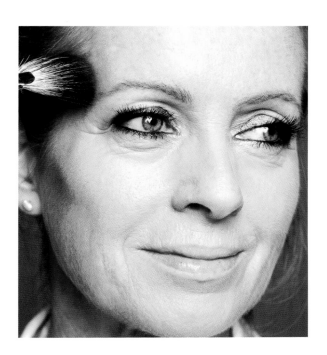

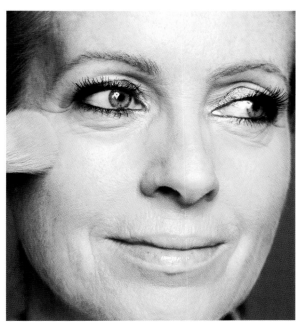

3 I have contoured underneath Sarah's cheekbones to enhance her cheeks (see the Contouring chapter on page 162). To do this I have used a brush that is no wider than my pinky finger. I have chosen a skin tone colour that is five shades darker than Sarah's natural skin tone and matt in texture.

4 A great technique for women with a high forehead or fine hair is to shade around the hairline to achieve a softer, more contoured look. I have applied a stronger amount on the temple area to achieve a more rounded forehead that is softer in shape and that also lifts the eyes and defines the cheekbones.

TIP

If you don't have the right product for contouring handy, you can use eye shadows that are dark brown and matt in texture. Eyebrow eye shadows are great for this.

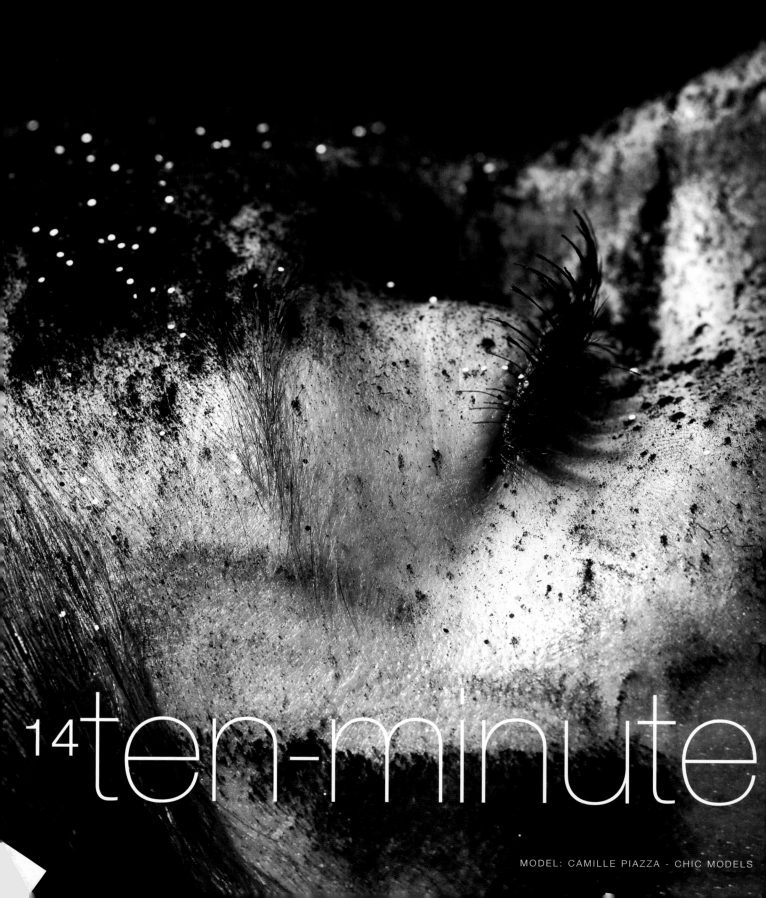

¹⁴ten-minute

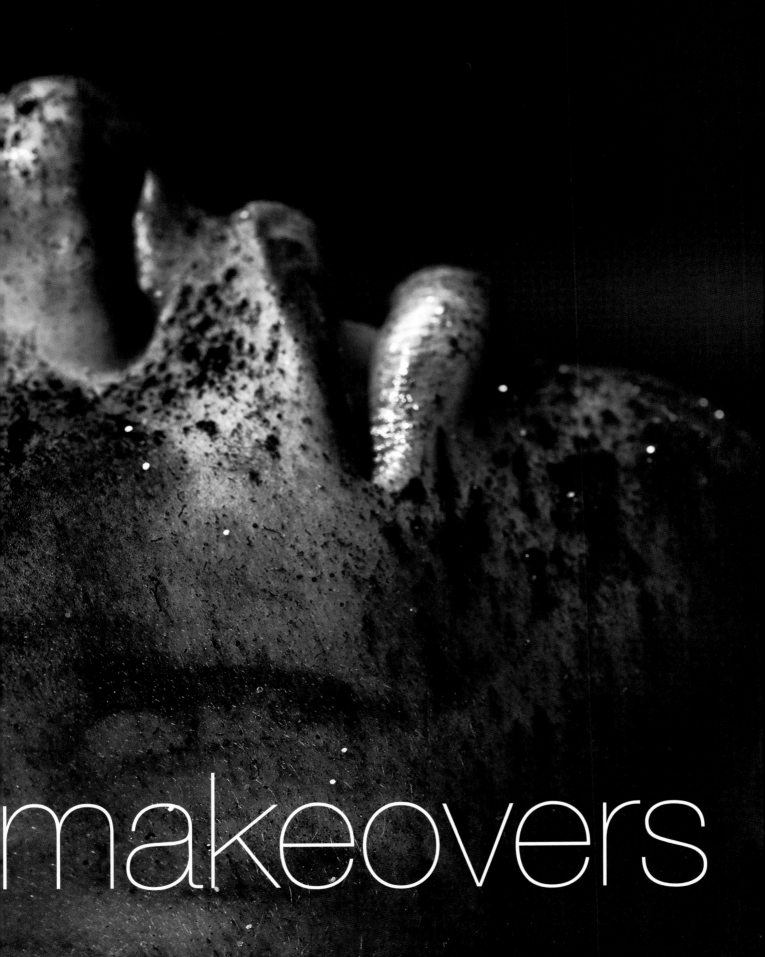

makeovers

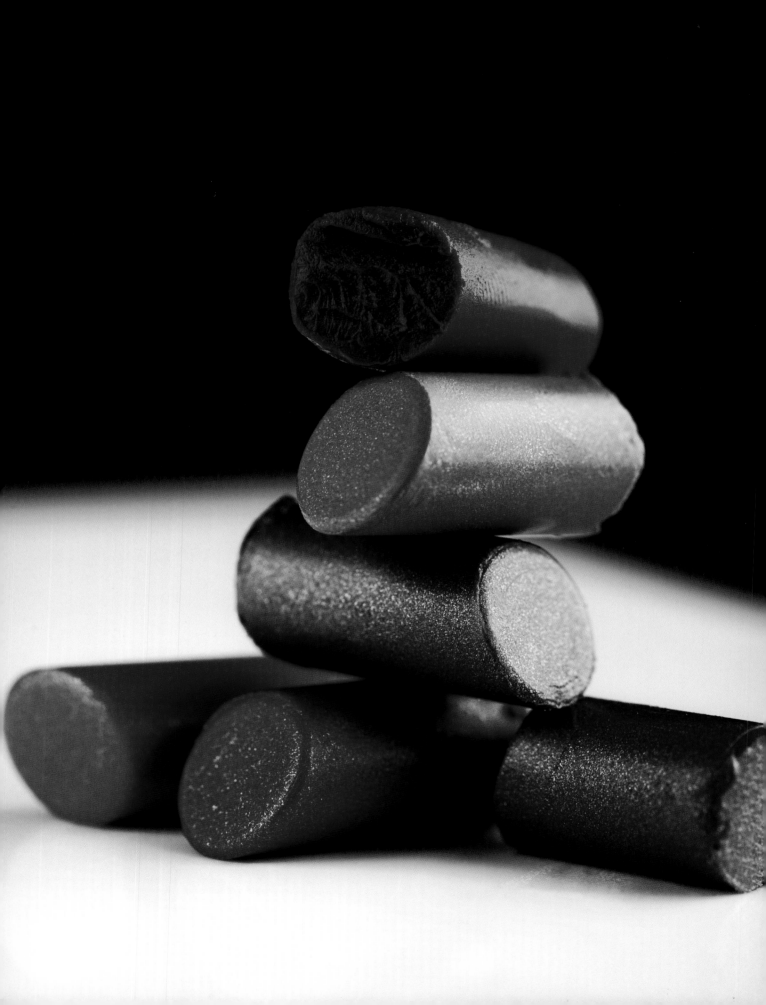

W ell, this chapter needs no introduction; the title speaks for itself. But what the hell … Much of the makeup you see in this book takes longer than 10 minutes, and takes more than a single attempt to get it right. And if you're like me and have no patience at all, you may want to start here before commencing some of the more difficult makeup in the Eyes chapter.

All the makeup in this chapter takes minimal time and expertise. Some of the looks are perfect as a way of transforming your day makeup into a sexy evening look, or simply a great way to look fabulous in minutes when you have to race out the door for work in the morning.

One of my best tips for applying makeup with 'no time' is to do your eyes first, because you can always do your foundation in the car at stop lights, or on the bus (people will just think you're applying moisturiser or sunscreen), or in the bathroom at work just before you have to enter the office. Remember, your eyes take the longest and need the most precision, so it makes sense to do what's hardest first!

However, in this chapter you will find easy, foolproof ways of doing your makeup quickly. It helps to refer to the Eye Colour Charts chapter (page 42) to make sure you're using the right colours to enhance your eyes.

General tips for doing your makeup in a hurry

- Don't go for makeup that is too complicated, such as liquid eyeliner and false eyelashes, as these take time and accuracy.
- Opt for products that you can smudge and blend. Avoid pencils and paints that are waterproof because they can't be easily repaired if you make a mistake (you'll have to remove them completely and start again).
- Know your accent colours (see the Eye Colour Charts chapter on page 42). These are colours that make your eyes look amazing and take only seconds to apply.
- If you like minimal eye makeup but love strong lips, then do your foundation first because it's difficult to blend foundation around a strong lip colour.
- If you are using shimmery eye shadow, don't apply mascara until after all of the shimmery shadow has been applied, as any fallout on the lashes tends to look like dandruff.
- And remember, no matter how much of a hurry you are in, your foundation must be blended well.

soft silver day look

This is a slightly wet look without the risk of it creasing and is a great way to give your eyelids a high sheen (wet eyelids never last for more than 5 minutes and are completely impractical). You can get the same effect by using soft, glittery eye shadows. This is a great look that is easy to achieve. It's also one of the only looks you can do with your fingers.

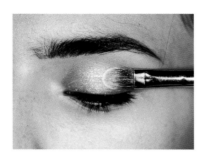

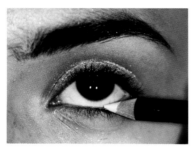

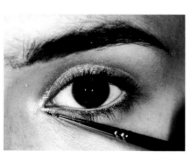

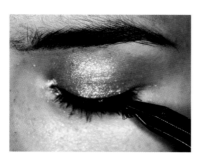

1 Using a small brush, apply a fine glittery pigment to the eyelid. Because this pigment is more glittery than normal eye shadow, it can also be used on the cheeks as more of a soft diamond effect than a frost.

2 Apply a creamy white pencil to the inner rim of the eye. Note the pencil is more of an eggshell white. Concealer pencils are great for this because they have more of a skin tone. This enlarges the eyes and wakens tired eyes (which is useful after a big night out).

3 Using a wet, very fine brush, apply the same colour you used on the lid to the inner corner of the eye. This adds that wow-factor and gives the eyes extra sparkle. (This is great for eyes that are closely set.)

4 Apply black mascara to the top lashes only, but if you want to make your eye shape more rounded, apply to the top and bottom. Use single false lashes and apply heavily to the top lid.

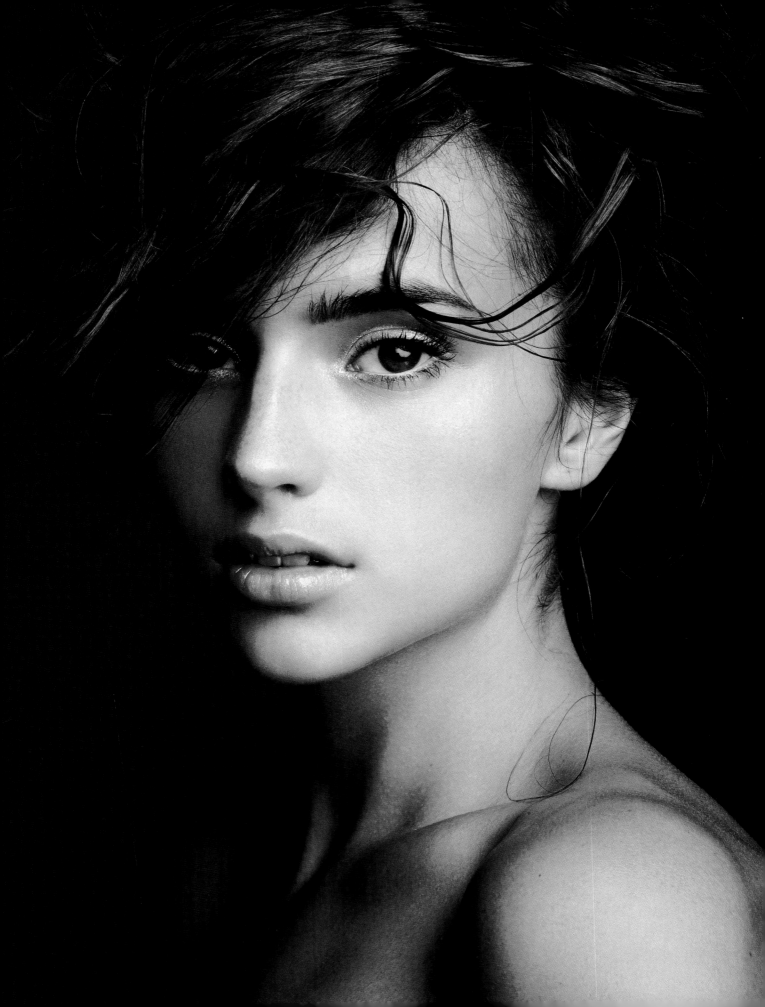

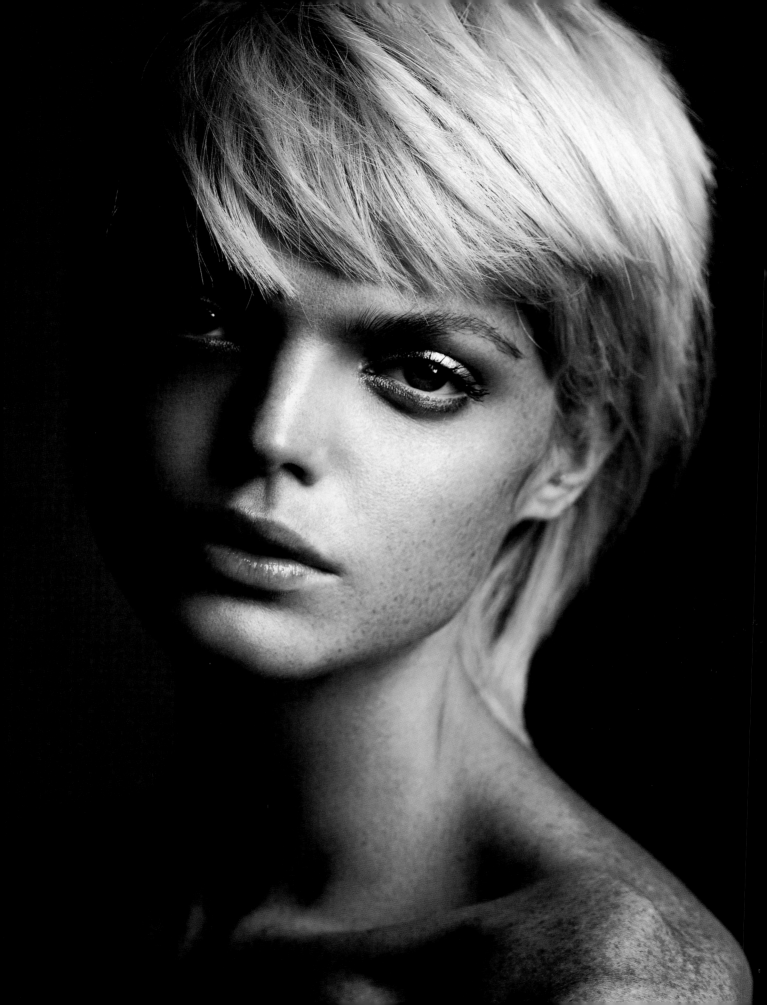

metallic day look

1 Prep the eyes and lightly apply foundation. Using a wet small brush, apply a strong silver pigment all the way across the lid, stopping just under the brow bone.

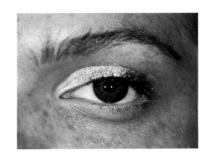

2 Using a wet thin brush, apply an antique gold pigment under the eye, close to the lash line.

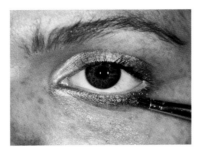

TIPS

It is very important to do the mascara only when you are completely happy with the eye shadow because of the fallout.

I have a 'thing' for shiny eyebrows! So I use a little clear lip gloss; it's also great for keeping your brows in place.

3 Apply a creamy white pencil to the inner rim of the eye. This is great for tired eyes as it will open them up and make them look brighter.

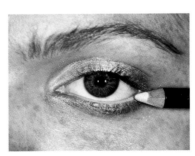

4 Curl lashes, and apply black mascara to the top lashes only. Use a cream blush to make the skin look dewy (this also refreshes tired-looking eyes). Apply a berry lip stain to the lips and eyebrows (optional).

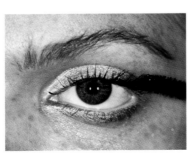

earthy tones

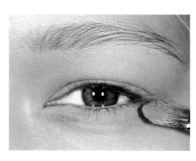

1 Lightly powder the lids for easier blending. Then, using a medium brush, apply a soft wash of terracotta eye shadow around the eye (on the whole eyelid up to the brow bone, and under the bottom lashes).

TIP

For step 4, if you have smaller eyes you can cheat a little and lift the contour shape slightly above; this creates the illusion of bigger eyelids.

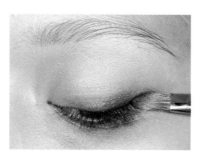

2 Twist the brush side on to give it a narrower edge, and apply a matt mahogany-brown shadow to the lash line. Keep it extra close to the lash line, as you want this colour to blend out to the terracotta.

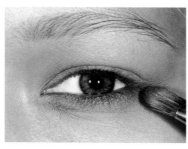

3 Apply the same mahogany shadow to the outside edge of the top lid. Remember, if the shadow drops under the eye, you can clean it up afterwards just before applying foundation. Notice I'm using a smaller brush now and keeping the colour close to the lash line.

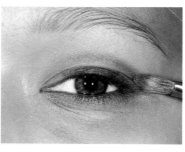

4 To create more depth to the eye, looking straight ahead and using the same brush, follow the shape of your lash line with the mahogany shadow, under the brow bone, keeping the outer edge (where the brush is in the picture) as the darkest point.

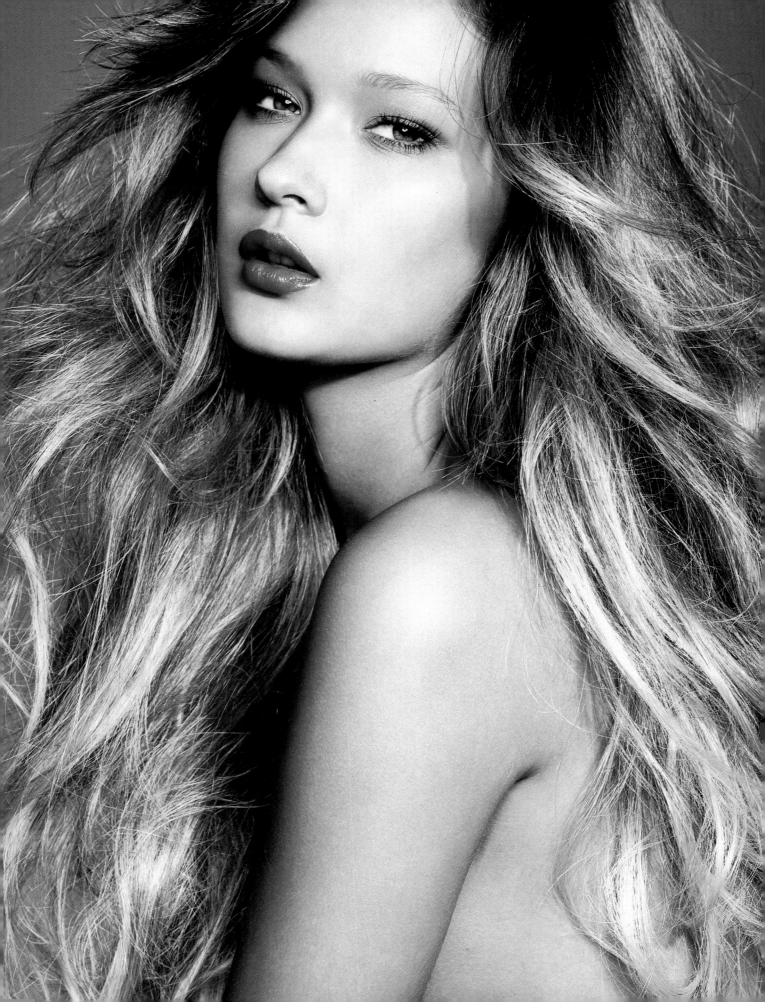

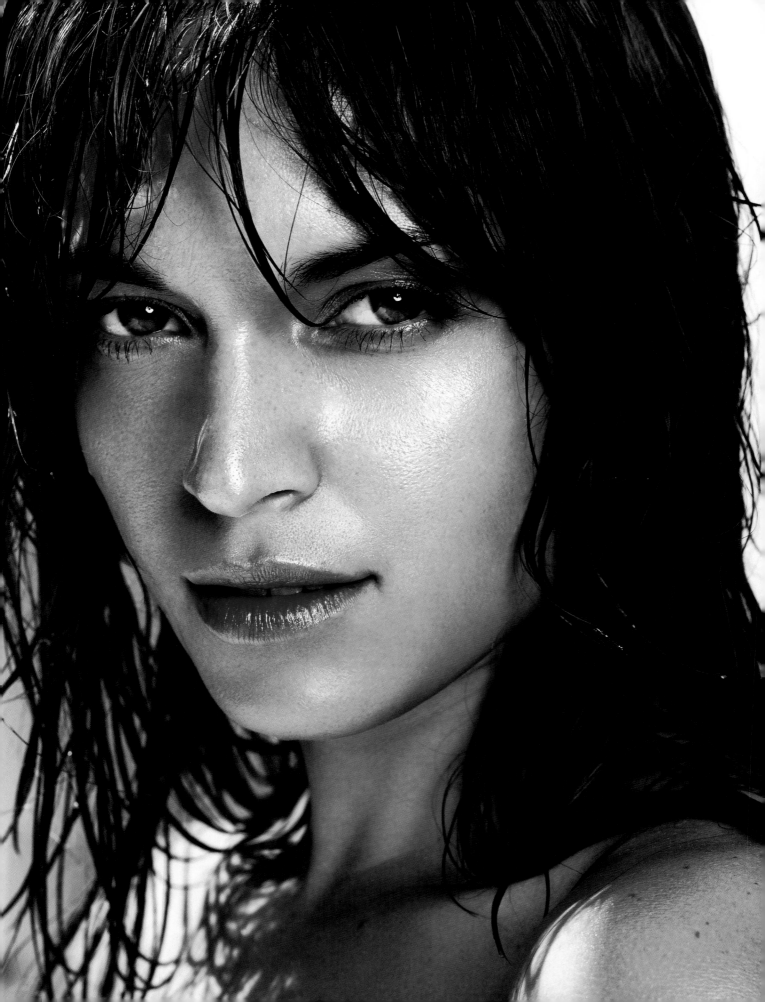

beach makeup

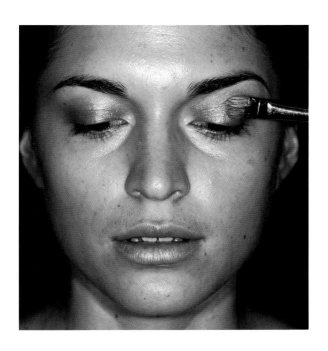 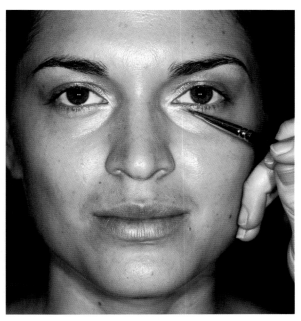

1 As you know, grease foundations and eye colours crease very easily. In this shot, we are using a grease-based cheek colour on the eyelids. You can also use lipstick as blush and eye colour. The good thing about grease-based products is that they are waterproof. The eyelids need to be stretched to apply the colour. This is another occasion when you can use your fingers to apply. I chose a metallic, high-shine golden bronze.

2 Using a very fine brush, apply a cream-textured highlighter colour or grease-based eye shadow heavily to the inner corners of the eyes. Grease eye shadows will crease, but they are the best for outdoors as you can just smooth away the creases instead of carrying around makeup brushes with you on the beach.

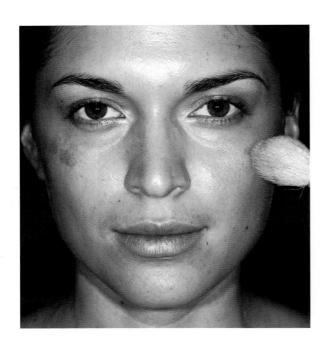

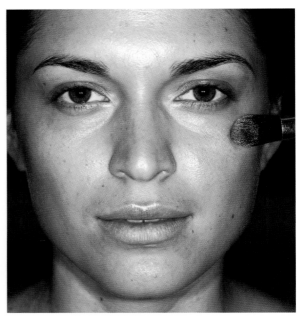

3 Apply a grease-based blush to the cheeks; this is great for that sun-kissed look. To blend, use a kabuki brush with circular motions. Grease blushes move around because of the grease, but can be easily smoothed back into the skin, making them perfect for outdoor use.

4 Apply a gold grease-based highlighter all over the face (see the Highlighting chapter on pages 196–202). Finish the look by applying a lip stain on the mouth. Lip stain is good for the beach as it is transparent. (It is unpleasant to see thick lipstick on someone at the beach, plus it's too sticky.)

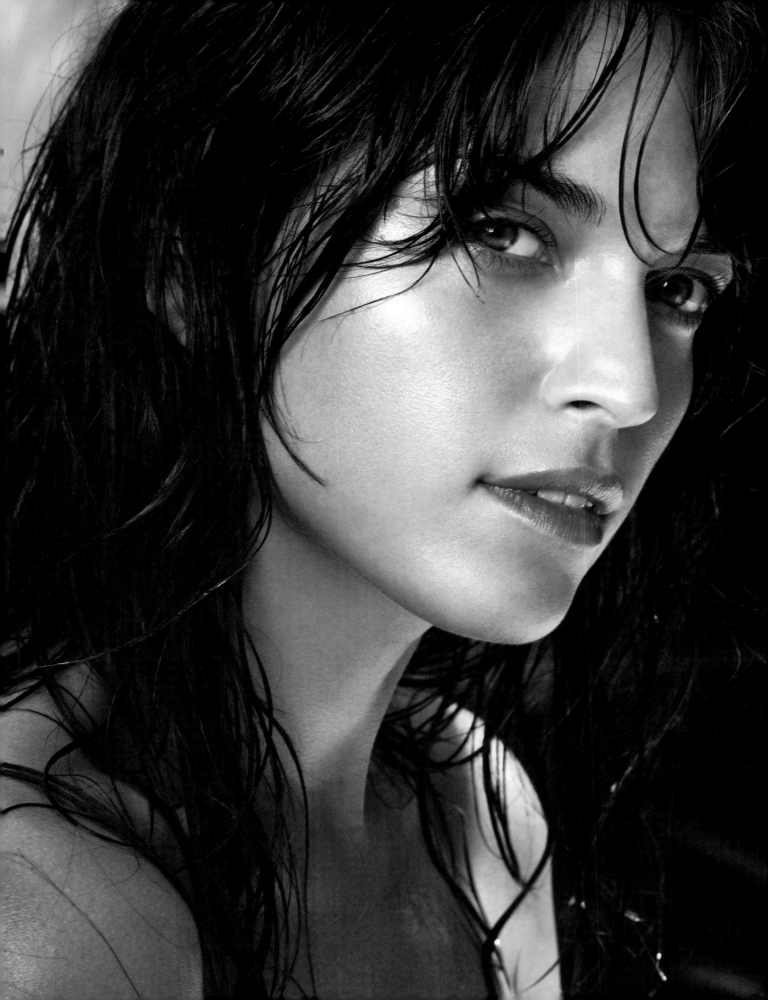

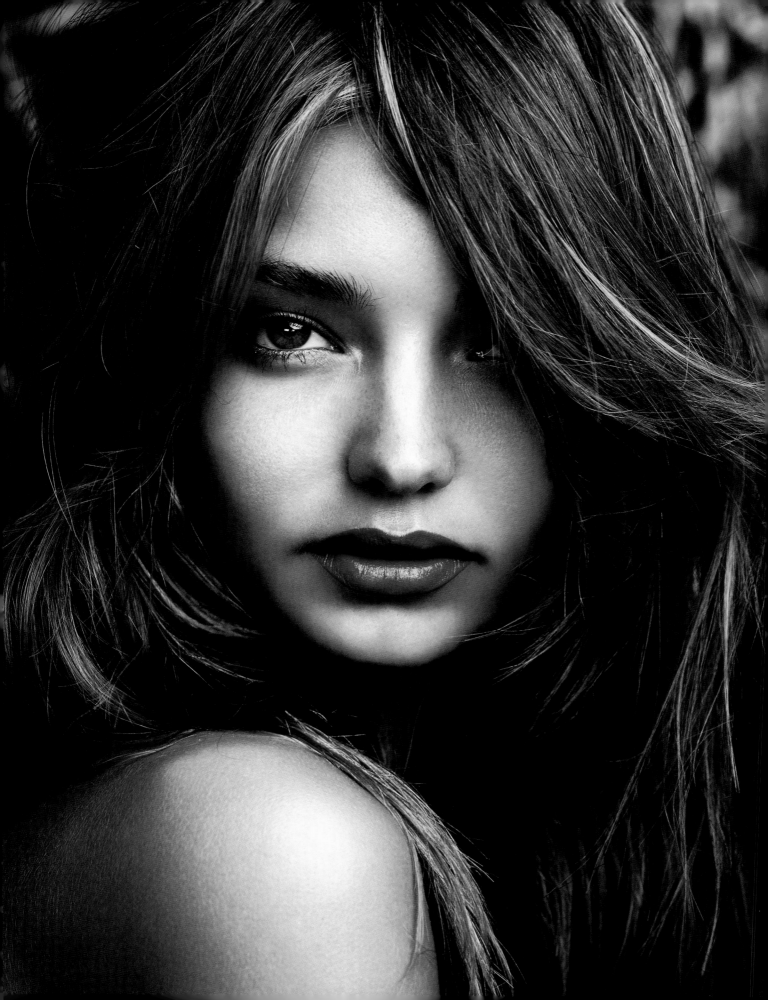

natural look

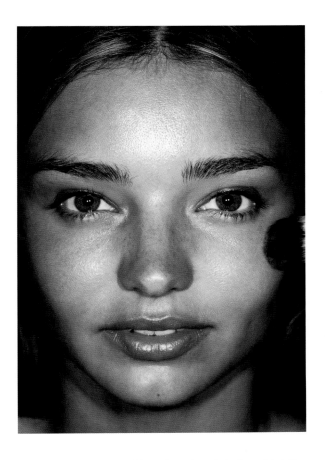 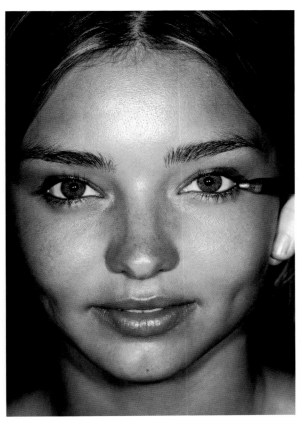

1 Apply sunscreen with a tinted moisturiser. Lightly conceal under the eyes, then apply a rose-coloured cheek stain. Remember to apply and blend quickly, otherwise it will stain in places you don't want it to.

2 Apply a heavy gold non-waterproof eyeliner to the inner rim of the eye. Remember, your inner eye is moist so waterproof pencils just won't work.

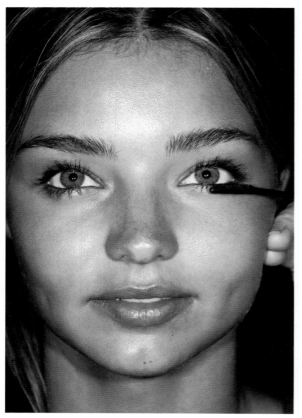

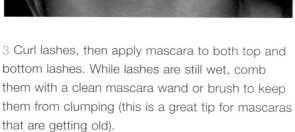

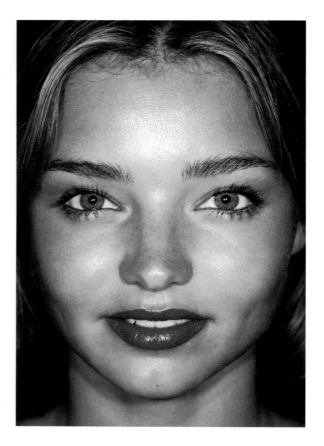

3 Curl lashes, then apply mascara to both top and bottom lashes. While lashes are still wet, comb them with a clean mascara wand or brush to keep them from clumping (this is a great tip for mascaras that are getting old).

4 Finish by applying red lipstick. Because Miranda has blue eyes, I am using an orange-based red. Usually, I would go for a blue-based red, but to make blue eyes stand out, the orange base is best.

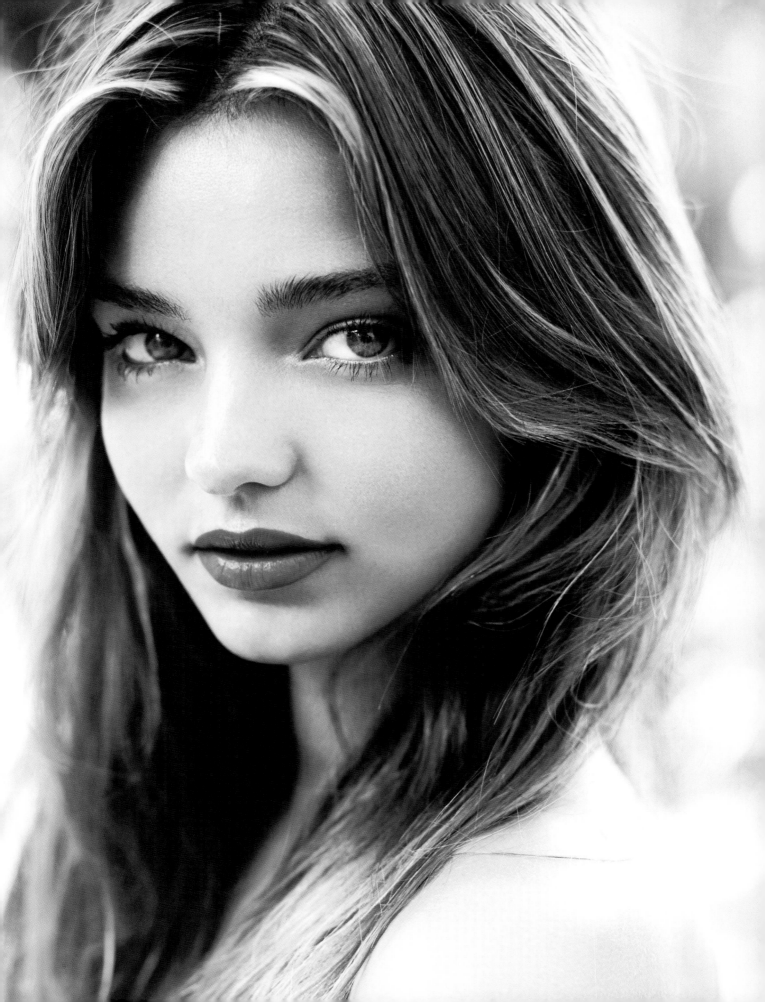

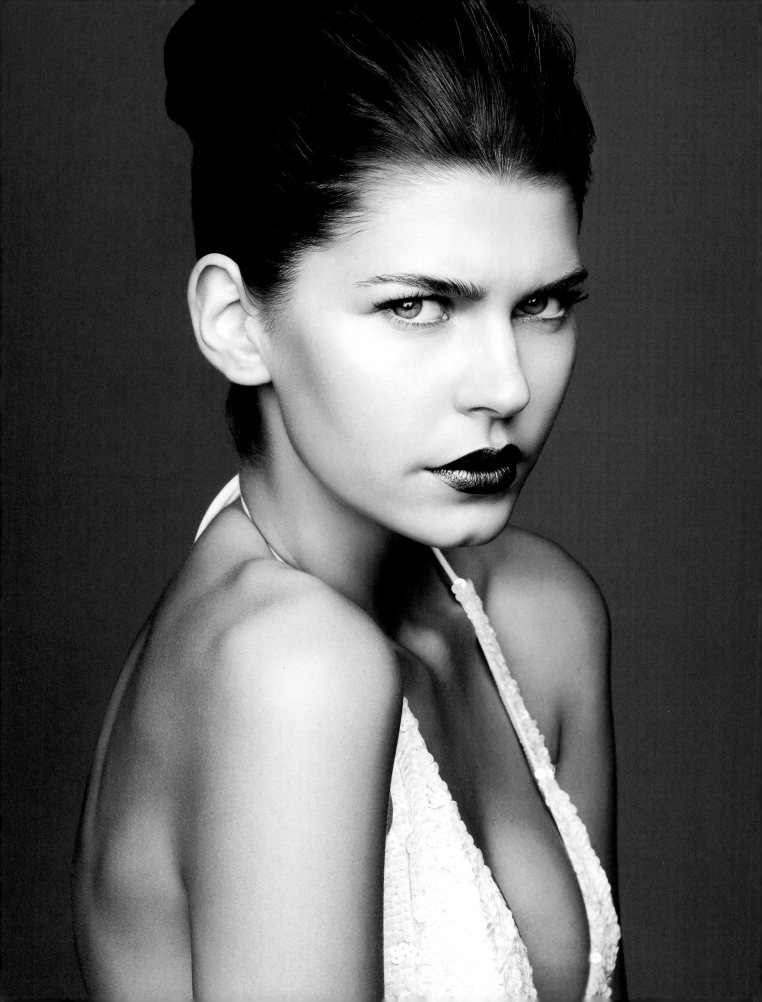

dramatic evening look

1 Using a fibre-optic brush, apply a sheer liquid foundation to the whole face. I have added a liquid illuminiser to give the skin extra glow—just add a few drops in with your foundation and use your brush to mix (do not do this if the skin is blemished, extremely oily or heavily sun-damaged).

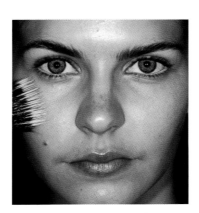

2 Apply a pink-gold cream blush with your fingers to the cheeks and to the cupid's bow of the lips. Then using a medium brush, apply the blush to the eyelids. This is one of those rare occasions where you can also use your fingers to do this.

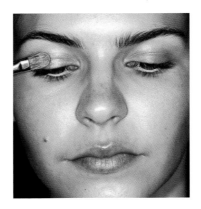

TIP

As cream eye colours crease very easily, you have to constantly smooth out the creases that your eye naturally has.

3 Put clear lip gloss on a clean mascara wand or brow brush and apply to the eyebrows—it holds them in place and gives them a sexy shine. Finish by applying a strong purple metallic lipstick to your lips with a lip brush.

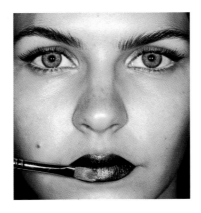

the morning after

For this shot, I wanted to show what you can do with heavy makeup from the night before. We had done a shoot with our model Cassie using heavy black eyes. I gave her strict instructions not to take her eye makeup off, and asked her to go to bed and to see me bright and early the next morning. The best thing about having a big night where you can't get all your makeup off is that you are always left with a perfect eyeliner around your eyes. So, the next day, Cassie came in with black panda eyes, looking as though she had been in a boxing ring with Muhammad Ali. And our ten-minute makeover could begin!

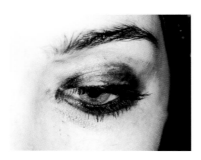

1 In this shot, you can see how heavy the makeup was around the eyes.

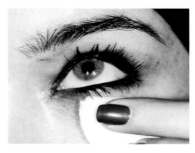

2 Remove as much of the black from your upper and lower lids as possible. Make sure you use a non-oily makeup remover, as this allows foundation to be directly applied after makeup removal. Oily removers require full cleansing of the face before makeup application.

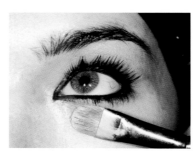

3 Using a medium brush, reapply foundation to the eyelids, and underneath the eyes.

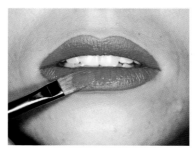

4 Finish by applying lipstick. In this case, I used the brightest orange lipstick I could find—perfect for making blue eyes really pop!

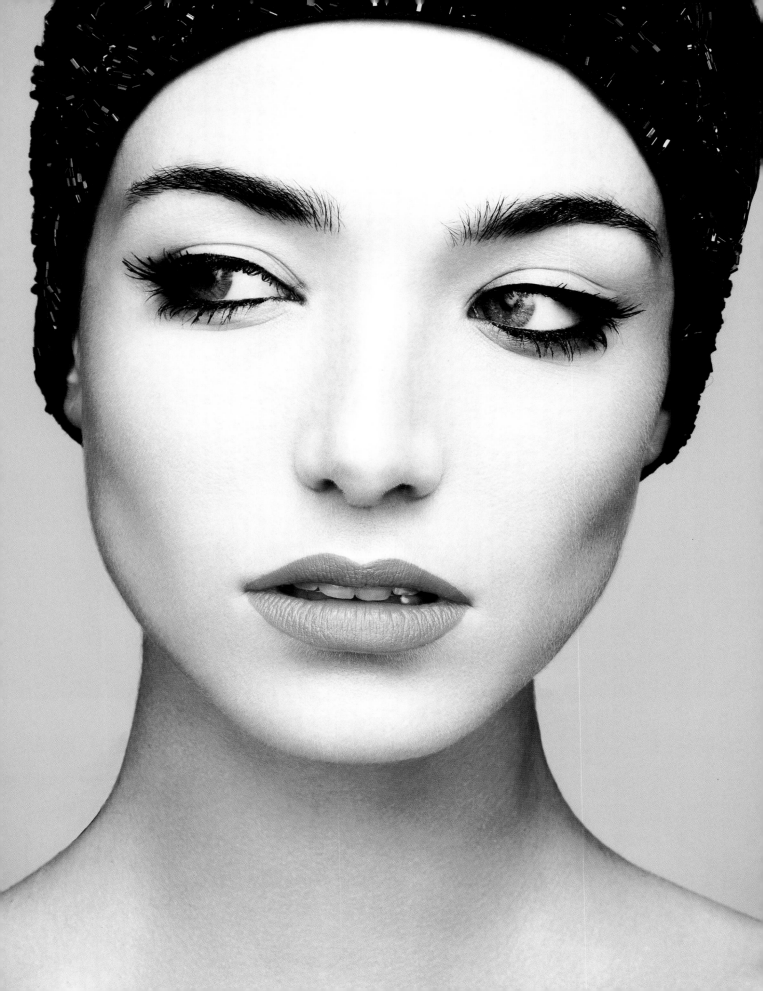

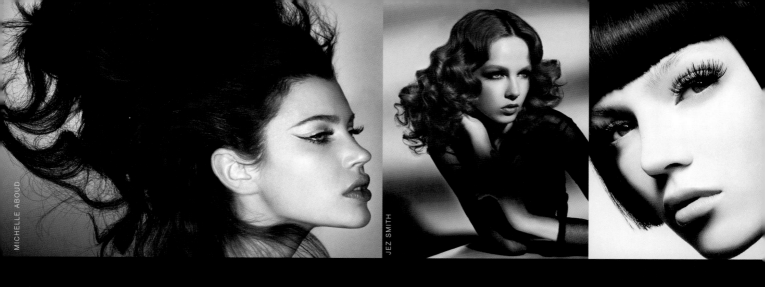

MICHELLE ABOUD

JEZ SMITH

RAE'S GALLERY

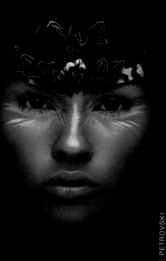

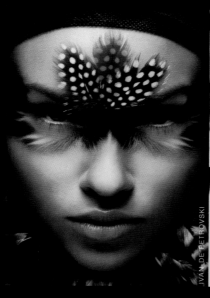

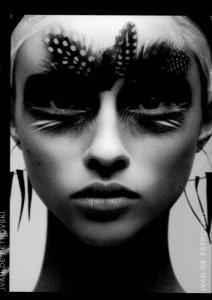

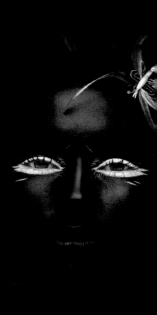

IVAN DE PETROVSKI

IVAN DE PETROVSKI

IVAN DE PETROVSKI

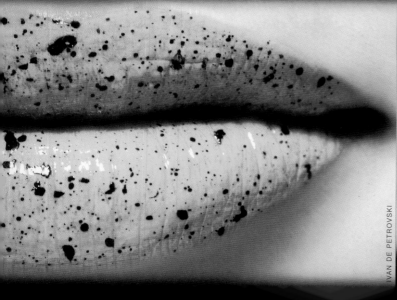

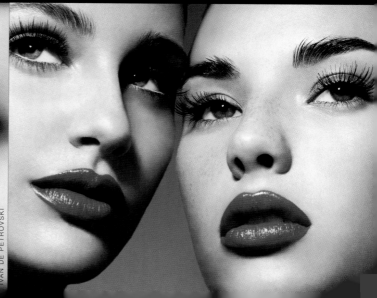

IVAN DE PETROVSKI

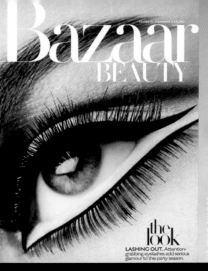

Bazaar
BEAUTY

the look

HOT LIPS. Slick your lips red, the sexiest colour in the spectrum.

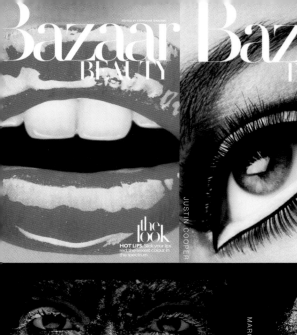

Bazaar
BEAUTY

the look

LASHING OUT. Attention-grabbing eyelashes add serious glamour to the party season.

JUSTIN COOPER

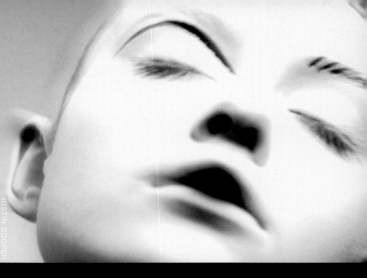

JUSTIN COOPER

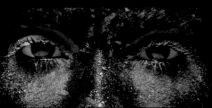

MARC DEBNAM

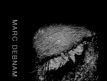

MARC DEBNAM

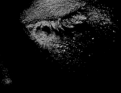

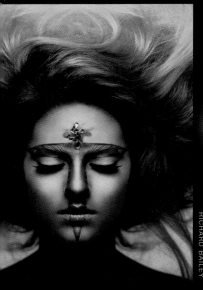

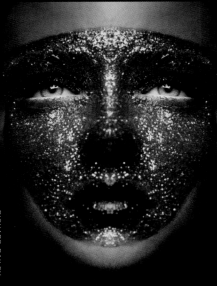

RICHARD BAILEY

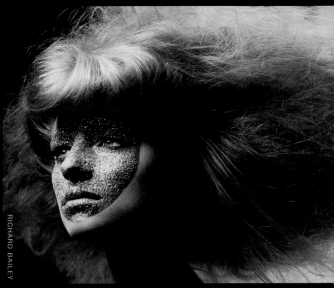

RICHARD BAILEY

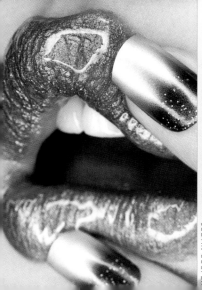

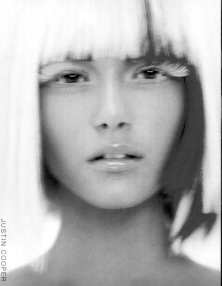

JUSTIN COOPER

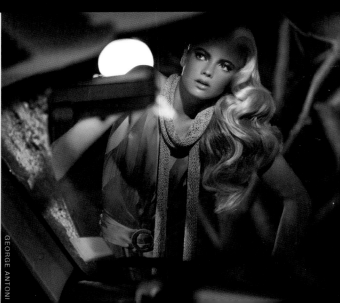

GEORGE ANTONI

246

index